MARRIAGE
MADE ME
FAT!

BOOK YOUR PLACE ON OUR WEBSITE AND MAKE THE READING CONNECTION!

We've created a customized website just for our very special readers, where you can get the inside scoop on everything that's going on with Zebra, Pinnacle and Kensington books.

When you come online, you'll have the exciting opportunity to:

- View covers of upcoming books
- Read sample chapters
- Learn about our future publishing schedule (listed by publication month *and author*)
- Find out when your favorite authors will be visiting a city near you
- Search for and order backlist books from our online catalog
- Check out author bios and background information
- Send e-mail to your favorite authors
- Meet the Kensington staff online
- Join us in weekly chats with authors, readers and other guests
- Get writing guidelines
- AND MUCH MORE!

**Visit our website at
http://www.kensingtonbooks.com**

MARRIAGE
MADE ME
FAT!

Understand Your Weight Gain— and Lose Pounds Permanently

EDWARD ABRAMSON, Ph.D.
Author of *Emotional Eating*

KENSINGTON BOOKS
KENSINGTON PUBLISHING CORP.
http://www.kensingtonbooks.com

KENSINGTON BOOKS are published by

Kensington Publishing Corp.
850 Third Avenue
New York, NY 10022

First Kensington Hardcover Printing: June, 1999
First Kensington Paperback Printing: May, 2000
10 9 8 7 6 5 4 3 2 1

Printed in the United States of America

For Anne and Jeremy,
and for Crystal

Contents

Acknowledgments

My interest in marriage and weight started more than fifteen years ago when I was directing a weight-loss program at a local hospital. In our weekly group meetings, many of the women described the difficulties they experienced with their husbands as they started losing weight. A lucky few reported that their husbands were encouraging and showed interest in the changes they were making. I am indebted to all of these women for sharing their experiences and helping me appreciate the role that weight plays in marital relationships. Some of their stories, with the identifying characteristics changed, appear in this book.

Many people have contributed, in one way or another, to the writing of this book. Early in my career, Dr. Richard Wunderlich introduced me to the joys (and frustrations) of conducting research on obesity and weight loss. Drs. Sara Armstrong, B. Gordon Gibb, Paul Spear, Marv Megibow, and Jane Rysberg have been supportive throughout my career at Chico State. When I had the idea to write a book on weight and marriage, Lynn Rosen of the Leap First Literary Agency encouraged me to develop it, then patiently guided me through several revisions until a workable proposal emerged. I enjoyed her calls, notes, and e-mails even when the message was that I should do again whatever I had just done. Tracy Bernstein, my editor at Kensington, was able to find the right mixture of humor, support, and gentle prodding so that I didn't stray too far from the next deadline. My friends and Bodega Bay neighbors, Suzanne Cushman and Noel Barnhurst, listened and offered support and encouragement. Dana Powers and Christine Thomas, two graduate students at Chico State, did their thesis research in this area. I benefited from their thorough research reviews. Christine, a former manager of a commercial weight-loss program, read many of the chapters and gave me feedback from the perspective of her clients.

The second half of this book was written while I was on sabbatical leave at the Division of Psychiatry and Psychology, United Medical and Dental Schools—University of London. I am indebted to several people who made the leave possible. In London Prof. Jim Watson and Dr. Bernard Rosen arranged my appointment at U.M.D.S., while Dr. Marv Megibow helped with arrangements on the Chico end. My daughter, Anne, took care of business while I was gone, while my son, Jeremy, helped every time I got into trouble with my computer. Finally, I want to express my appreciation to my wife, Crystal. She gave me support throughout, listened patiently to whatever problem I was trying to solve, and often suggested alternative wordings when I got stuck. I am also grateful that she did not gain any weight while I was preoccupied with writing and was less available to be a nurturing husband.

Introduction

The Internet has hundreds of newsgroups where complete strangers use their computers to discuss topics of mutual interest. On an Internet support group for dieters Kathleen posted a question:

"Hi! I'm new to this group. Maybe somebody can shed some light on a topic. When I was single I weighed a lot less. But now that I've settled down with someone I have blossomed! Does this happen with a lot of people, or is it just me?" Within hours the Information Superhighway was buzzing with similar tales.

Sandy responded, "I don't know if this happens to many of us, but when I got married I gained a lot of weight. He cooked the most marvelous but highly fattening foods. It was just so easy to not worry about it. Since we also went out to eat frequently, it made the problem worse."

Rosemary, a dieter from England, showed that relationships can affect weight on both sides of the Atlantic. She said, "I wanted to spend time with my boyfriend and because I had so little time, I gave up exercising, which wasn't a good idea. We broke up (not because of food or weight) and I've lost 40 pounds since then. I think your significant other's eating habits contribute to your lifestyle."

Joan contributed her experience: "My husband is a compulsive eater, and I'm following him. I notice when I am not around him, when he's taken a trip alone, I'm able to control my eating at home and actually lose. But when he comes back, I go right back to eating in his style. Help. How do I maintain myself when around him, and not buy into his eating habits?"

Kathleen, Sandy, Rosemary, and Joan described a few of the weight-producing changes that come with marriage, or sometimes with long-term relationships. For most women, the process is not as obvious as having a husband who is a gourmet cook or a compulsive eater. Even if your husband is thin and hates to cook, getting married can produce many subtle changes in your eating habits. In most marriages, the changes are not sudden or dramatic; they evolve over the years. This book will help you understand the changes that come with marriage, and show you how to use your marriage for weight reduction rather than weight gain.

Marriage Is Fattening

Your lifestyle changed after you got married. Many of these changes added pounds. If you have children, there were more changes to your daily routine and additional pounds. These pounds, and more importantly, how you feel about them, become part of the relationship you have with your husband. For many women, being married helped to make them fat and prevented them from losing weight despite their best efforts.

I am not suggesting that your weight gain was the result of a deliberate plot on the part of your husband. He will probably be just as surprised as you are when he recognizes how pound-producing rituals and patterns have developed. Without assigning blame, he can become an ally in reversing these rituals and patterns. Part I—"Is Your Marriage Making You Fat?"—will help you identify the role being married has played in your weight gain.

Most husbands don't view eating the same way as their wife does. You know that food is more than just the fuel that makes your body run. You know that eating is tied into your feelings, and often food substitutes for love. Chapter 1 describes how this works. You also know that your weight isn't determined by a single factor. Even though your husband may be involved, there are biological and social forces contributing to your weight gain. Chapters 2 and 3 describe eight reasons for weight gain and help you determine which are the most significant for you.

Chapter 4 provides the groundwork for "A Recipe for Losing Weight and Improving Your Relationship." The constructive role your husband can play will be described, along with practical methods for communicating with him about this sensitive issue. Chapter 4 also includes a letter to your husband explaining the Recipe and showing him why he will benefit from participating. Although it would be helpful, his cooperation is not essential. If your husband chooses not to participate, you will learn how to disengage your weight from the marital dynamics. When this has been accomplished, you will have fewer conflicts about eating and you'll find weight loss to be more straightforward.

Marriage Can Be Slimming

The Recipe is presented in Part II. It will help you clear the path for permanent weight loss by removing the barriers that interfered with your previous diets. You will learn a new way of thinking about dieting so that you can be good to yourself as you untie the knot between food and love. A brief questionnaire will help you assess the possible sexual consequences of your weight so that you can calm the fears that often hinder weight loss. You will examine your motivations and expectations for weight loss, and then go through a realistic goal-setting process that will set you up for success.

If your husband is going to be involved, you can show him the "Note for Your Husband" in several of the chapters. These explain what you are trying to accomplish and how he can help. For example, in Chapter 9 you will see if some of your eating is a means of suppressing anger or soothing yourself after an angry outburst. Instead of using food, you will learn to be constructively annoyed. Both of you will follow an eight-step sequence for resolving annoyance without angry outbursts or eating.

Instead of telling you to eat less and exercise more, the Recipe will offer specific methods for your husband to help increase your motivation and decrease the feelings of deprivation. You will be more comfortable reducing your fat consumption while increasing your activity level. The last chapter prepares you to deal with the potential detours that can derail the most ardent dieter. When you and your husband can identify difficult situations before they occur, you will have the tools to minimize their impact.

The Recipe may not be appropriate for everyone. If you are pregnant, lactating, or have significant medical problems, like diabetes or cardiovascular disease, you should seek medical advice before starting any weight reduction program. If you are bulimic or think that you might be anorexic, consult a competent psychologist or psychiatrist. Finally, if your marriage has deteriorated to the point that you are seriously considering divorce, this would not be a good time to start the Recipe. Several of the methods will change aspects of your relationship with your husband. If either of you have a tenuous commitment to your marriage, it may not be strong enough to withstand these alterations. It would be better to seek marriage counseling first, to put your marriage on a stronger footing, and then work on the Recipe. On the other hand, if the two of you squabble, or you're just going through a period of marital blahs, don't be scared off. The Recipe will help you lose weight *and* improve your relationship.

PART I

Is Your Marriage Making You Fat?

CHAPTER 1

Why Food Substitutes for Love

Men eat because their stomachs growl. Men eat because it is noon, and time for lunch. Men eat because the waitress wheels the dessert cart to the table and the chocolate mousse cake looks great. Women eat for all these reasons, and one more: because they don't feel loved. Many women use food for comfort when they are lonely or their romantic relationship is unsatisfying.

Your struggle with weight and diet doesn't make any sense to your husband. His experience is different. He can afford to be detached and logical about dieting; his whole worth as a human being isn't tied up in the number that emerges when he steps on the scale. Even if he's gained a few pounds, your husband is worthwhile because of his career, his ability to provide for his family, his charming personality, and the corny jokes that he tells. On the other hand, even if you have an equally worthwhile career, make more money, and tell better jokes, you still feel bad if the scale shows an increase from the last time you checked.

Food, eating, weight, and dieting are different for women than they are for men. While both sexes can agree on the tangible aspects, when it comes to the subjective meanings and emotional connotations, men and women can't begin to communicate. Take a lowly french fry, for example. You could have a discussion with your husband about the relative merits of McDonald's vs. Burger King's french fries, how much salt is desirable, and even how many grams of fat there are in a single fry, but if french fries are on your list of forbidden foods, would he understand how bad you feel if you eat a few? Those french fries have an emotional significance far beyond their caloric value. Katherine, a 32-year-old mother of two, contrasted her experience eating forbidden foods with her husband's:

> When Todd wants some ice cream he marches over to the refrigerator and helps himself to a huge bowl. If I tease him about getting fat, he makes a joke and goes right on eating. When I eat something that isn't on my diet I feel so guilty. Usually I try to sneak the food when I'm by myself. If I get caught, I'm embarrassed. Even if he doesn't say anything I make an excuse or apologize. Why is it okay for him to eat whatever he wants, but it's not okay for me?

Love Handles vs. Cellulite

If your husband has seen his twenty-fifth birthday, it's unlikely that he still has a flat, "washboard" stomach (if he ever did). Maybe he laments having gained weight. Maybe he is nostalgic about his youth when he was more active, or maybe he just jokes about his beer belly, but do you ever get the feeling that his whole day is ruined because his pants are too tight? Compare his attitude with your feelings the first time you discovered dimpled flesh where you sit ("cellulite"). Since his experience is so different, it is very hard for him to understand how you feel when you look at your body in a mirror.

Why are men and women so different when it comes to food, weight, and diets? It's not some peculiar character-istic of you or your husband. Many studies have shown that American women are more concerned about their weight and what they eat. Women diet more often than men do, they check their weight more frequently, and they are more self-conscious about what they eat when others are around.[1]

Your physiology may contribute to your weight con-sciousness. Most likely your weight fluctuates more than your husband's, probably because of fluid changes associ-ated with menstruation. If his weight doesn't change as much as yours does, there is less reason for him to check it. Still, most weight consciousness comes from social influences. Just go to the movies, turn on the TV, or look at ads in fashion magazines. The message is clear—attractive women are slim. Don't you want to be attractive too?

Despite more than 30 years of feminism, appearance is still more important for women than it is for men, and your weight is an important part of your appearance. Look-ing good increases your popularity, gives you more status, and makes it more likely that you'll snag a desirable spouse. Whether it makes any sense or not, in our culture being thin is part of being attractive, but it's also more than that.

A slim, well-groomed, fashionably dressed woman con-veys a positive image even if her facial features don't rate a 10. By virtue of her thin physique, she is seen as competent, successful, and in control. Contrast this with a heavy woman, even if she has a stunningly beautiful face. Because she is overweight, she is seen as lazy and obviously self-indulgent. With so much depending on your weight, it's easy to understand why you are more concerned when you see dimples in your thighs than your husband is when his love handles blossom.

Illogical and Immoral

Since weight is not critical for most men, they have difficulty understanding the psychological significance it has for women. Men tend to see eating, weight, and dieting in either logical or moralistic terms. The male view is that if you think you are too fat, you should eat less, exercise more, or do some of both. This is the logical, straightforward solution to the problem. If, after having this solution explained to you, you still can't stick to your diet, it must be because you lack willpower (in other words, you are morally weak and lack self-discipline). Women know that it is never that simple. You may not be able to explain it, but with so much riding on your weight, you know that your husband's logical explanation is missing something. You understand as well as anyone else the connections between eating, exercise, and weight, so any weight you've gained isn't the result of ignorance.

What about your willpower? Is there a lack of willpower that makes it so hard for you to lose weight? Are those persistent pounds a result of some deep-seated personality defect that renders you unable to exercise self-discipline? Unlikely. Look at other parts of your life. If you're a mom, you make yourself get out of bed in the middle of the night to take care of your sick child. If you work outside of the home, there are mornings when the alarm rings that you want to roll over and go back to sleep, but you make yourself get up and go to work anyway. How about when you were in school? Can you remember forcing yourself to stay awake to finish the paper that was due the next morning? If you think about it, you can find many situations where you've demonstrated willpower and self-discipline, so why is losing weight so hard?

Feel Bad, Eat, Feel Worse, Repeat

If controlling your weight is so essential to your sense of well-being, and you are not lacking in willpower, why is it so difficult to lose weight? Many dieters report that they do pretty well until they experience food cravings. This is more than just liking a food, or a preference for one food over another. When you crave a food, it takes over your thinking; you become preoccupied with it. You may like other foods as much, but if you have a craving for chocolate, nothing else will do, and it's hard to do anything else until you've had your chocolate.

Emotions and craving and eating are all tied together for women. One review of research found that almost all overweight women eat to soothe unpleasant emotions like loneliness, depression, boredom, anxiety, and anger, while far fewer men used food for comfort.[2] For women who experience food cravings, a negative mood almost always precedes the craving.[3] Women are more likely than men to be emotional eaters and experience food cravings.

While women are more likely to experience food cravings, when men do have a craving, they are no better at resisting it than women are. The vast majority of men and women who experience cravings give in to them. When it comes to food cravings, both sexes have trouble with "willpower," but research shows that there are differences in feelings after eating. Most men feel good after satisfying their craving. They enjoyed eating the food that they craved and they felt good about having done it. Women, on the other hand, were much more likely to feel bad afterward.[4]

These findings help explain why it is so hard for many women to stick to their diets. For women, negative emotions produce food cravings. Food cravings inevitably result in eating food which isn't on your diet. (Did you ever crave celery?) After giving in to the craving, you feel guilty, sad, frustrated, or ashamed. Your husband is less likely to be on a diet, is less likely to be an emotional eater, and is less concerned about his weight in general. When he experiences a craving and gives in, it's no big deal.

Box 1. Resisting the Craving

The next time you are seized by the irresistible urge for chocolate (or whatever), pause for a moment. You can have the chocolate in a minute, but first ask yourself what you are feeling. Obviously you are feeling the craving, but what emotions are you experiencing? What did you feel before you started craving the food? Are you bored? Tense or stressed? Irritated or angry? Sad or lonely? See if you can find any feeling that is beneath the craving. Don't worry if you can't define it exactly. Just get a general sense of how you are feeling. Now, if you've got an idea of your feelings, the second step is to figure out why you feel this way. Did someone do something that hurt your feelings? Are you alone? Are you anticipating something in the near future that has you worried? Did someone treat you unfairly? Is there too much to do in too little time, or maybe today is a slow day with nothing interesting going on. See if you can identify what is going on that produced the emotion.

Why should you think about your emotional state? Because once the source of the emotion is clarified, the craving becomes less urgent. Since cravings usually last less than 12 minutes, if you decrease the urgency, it's easier to resist until the craving is gone. Now, if you still want the chocolate, go ahead and have some; just eat it slowly and make sure you enjoy it!

Don't gobble now and feel guilty later. When you aren't really enjoying it anymore, stop eating. You don't have to finish all of it. You can save the rest for another time when you would really enjoy it.

Craving Love

Many of the emotions that can produce cravings, especially loneliness and sadness, are related to problems with love and relationships. Francine, a 32-year-old computer programmer, is a good example of how this process works.

Francine lived alone in an upscale apartment complex. Since she frequently worked late, she'd stop at the neighborhood deli to pick up something for dinner. Francine was watching her weight so she was usually "good." She avoided fried or fatty foods, pulled the skin off the chicken she ate, and tried to fill up on vegetables and rice. After dinner, she would make a few phone calls, look through her mail, and then turn on the TV and flip through a magazine. Regardless of the program or the magazine article she was reading, after a few minutes a little thought would pop into her consciousness. She described the pattern to me:

At first it was harmless enough, just my curiosity asking, "I wonder if there are any peanut M&M's left." I'd dismiss the thought and go back to my reading, but it would come back a second time, only stronger and in more detail. "I knew I had some yesterday, did I finish them? Did I leave part of the bag in my dresser?" By this time I'm working hard, trying to forget about it, but it's no use. No matter what I try, I hear the M&M's calling me. I start visualizing the bag lying in the top drawer of my dresser. Pretty soon I'm up looking in the dresser. If I don't find the M&M's, I try to figure out where they might be. After searching for a minute or two, I conclude that there weren't any left over, I get my coat, and I'm off to 7-Eleven to buy a bag. By the time I'm back home, I've usually finished the whole thing. Then I feel miserable. I'm really down on myself. Each step of the way, I've been trying to ignore the craving. When that doesn't work, I try to talk myself out of it. I tell myself that if I eat the M&M's, I'm just going to feel guilty afterwards, but whatever logic I use doesn't work. It's like the M&M's have a magnetic pull that draws me to them.

Like most women, Francine's cravings were related to her feelings. We worked on tracking down the emotions that usually preceded her cravings. Almost always, it was a sad, lonely feeling.

Francine had never married but had had three long-term relationships since college. The first ended after her boyfriend entered a graduate program 1,500 miles away. Although they tried to maintain a long-distance relationship, after several months he became involved with an undergraduate at his new school. Her second relationship went on for six years, but eventually ended because he wanted to get married and have children. She knew that she wasn't ready for motherhood then, and couldn't promise him that she would change her mind in the near future. The third relationship never developed as far as the first two. After a year or so of off-and-on dating, Francine lost interest and broke it off. Each time, she knew intellectually that breaking up was the right thing to do, but she just couldn't get over the loneliness that followed. When she was involved in a relationship, the food cravings subsided. In between relationships, peanut M&M's exerted their magnetic pull.

Like Francine, many women with strong food cravings have told me that eating wasn't a deliberate attempt to console themselves when they were lonely, but rather they just found themselves craving something sweet, and the next thing they knew they were in the kitchen, standing in front of the refrigerator.

Most women are constantly preoccupied with their weight. When you are trying to avoid fattening foods, these forbidden foods become even more appealing. When you have been deprived of a desirable food, you may find yourself daydreaming about it, imagining how it will taste and visualizing yourself eating it. Then you have an emotional upset, or are just feeling a little blue and the craving for that food becomes stronger. If you are really motivated to stick to your diet, you may be able to resist the craving for a while, but usually, you give in. After eating the food you have been craving, do you feel better? Maybe for a few minutes, but then the guilt and self-recriminations set in. You feel bad all over again. For women, dieting and negative emotions produce food cravings which result in eating, which produces more bad feelings and stronger vows to diet tomorrow. Feeling bad about your eating, and ultimately about yourself, does *not* help weaken the cycle. Instead of feeling bad, understand how the cycle got started and then you will be able to work on changing your habits and lose weight. You can halt the "Feel bad, eat, feel worse" cycle.

The Roots of Cravings

It's easy to see why women are more concerned about weight than men are, but the special link between love and food for women is not so obvious. If you are a frequent food craver, you can identify with Francine's predicament. You're careful about what you eat. You know very well that the food you are craving is forbidden. You try to control yourself, yet sooner or later you will relent. The craving is too powerful. You are experiencing something too deeply rooted to be controlled by a little willpower. Before eating the first M&M, you know that the experience really won't be that great and you'll regret it afterward, yet the craving overrules logic. A force this powerful got its start early in life, before your very young brain was capable of logical thought. It has its roots in infancy, and developed through childhood and adolescence. The early linking of food and love is probably similar for boys and girls. A few years later, when sex role identity is established, girls' experiences strengthen the link while boys move on to other concerns.

Don't Feed, Sing

Since Freud, psychoanalysts have theorized that some disturbance during early infancy is responsible for later obesity. Although we now know that this is an oversimplification, that obesity can have many origins (see Chapters 2 and 3), early feeding experiences can lay the foundation for the food-love connection.

Imagine that you are an 8-month-old infant. Now, what's the scariest thing in the whole world? You haven't started worrying about Visa bills or your weight yet; the scariest thing is when your mother leaves you. Since you totally rely on her for everything, if she's gone, you're in deep trouble! If this wasn't bad enough, your 8-month-old mind has no way of knowing how long she will be gone when she steps out of the room. So when she leaves, you are lonely and terrified. When she comes back and finds you crying, she wants to comfort you. If she picks you up, cuddles you and sings to you, you feel better. Everything is fine; you feel secure and loved. If she picks you up but instead of singing she feeds you, you still feel better. Everything is fine, you are loved, but you have also learned an unfortunate lesson. You now associate eating with being comforted when you have scary feelings or are lonely.

Several decades later when you feel alone and unloved, what will you do? According to psychoanalysts, you'll eat. In one study, psychoanalysts reviewed their notes for 84 mostly female, obese patients. They found that weight gain was associated with feelings of being unloved or unwanted, and separations from others, more often than with other types of unconscious conflicts (like sex or aggression).[5] You don't have to be an ardent Freudian to see how early feeding experiences could lay the foundation for a pattern, later in life, where feeling lonely, unloved, or abandoned could cause a craving to eat. Still, if this was the only reason for the food-love connection, you'd probably be over it by now. Unfortunately, it isn't.

Family, Food, and Feelings

Think back to your elementary school days. Try to recall some of your happiest memories. If you can visualize that scene—take a mental snapshot of where you were, who you were with, and what was going on when you were a happy child. Was it one of your birthday parties? A Christmas or Thanksgiving family get-together? An especially close moment with one of your parents that made you feel warm and loved? Now if you have that scene fixed in your mind, look around and see if food is involved. Did your parents use food as a means of expressing their love for you? Look at the list of situations where food is paired with love, or just associated with being close to your parents to see how many fit for you:

- Celebrating a good report card or other accomplishment by going out for ice cream or another treat.
- Going out with your parents for pizza after an important game (sports) or recital (if you played an instrument).

- Receiving a "care package" from your parents when you went to summer camp or when you were living in the dorms at college.
- Your mother making chicken soup or another special food to help you recover when you were sick.
- Looking forward to sharing a special food that only you and your mother enjoyed.
- Your mother making a meal with your favorite foods to help celebrate an accomplishment or special occasion.
- Spending part of an afternoon in the kitchen with your mother making a special food or preparing an important meal.
- Your mother being especially proud of you when you learned to cook.

Food can be used to express love, but also the lack of love. Look at the list below and see if you recognize any instances where your parents may have been angry with you, or disappointed in you, and used food to express their negative feelings toward you:

- You were sent away from the table before you finished eating because you were "bad."
- You didn't get dessert because you didn't comply with a parental request.
- Your mother or father wouldn't let you leave the table until you had finished a food that you didn't like.
- A parent or sibling teased you about your food likes or dislikes.
- Your mother or father told you you'd never get married unless your cooking improved.

Starting in infancy, eating has been paired with love in your family. Then, as a young girl, you start experiencing expectations about your appearance. Since many of these expectations revolve around your weight, the basis for a lifelong conflict is being established: When you feel unloved, you eat to feel better, but this makes you less attractive, and therefore less lovable.

See Dick Run, See Jane Try on Mommy's Clothes

When you were young, you got countless messages, sometimes explicitly stated, other times just suggested, telling you that you had to look nice in order to be worthy of love. Try to remember fond memories from your childhood, times when you felt warm, secure, and loved. Most likely, your mom, dad, or grandparents were happy with you. They smiled, hugged you, and said nice things to you. What exactly did they say? What did you do to make them feel so loving toward you? Were you cute? Did they say you looked pretty? Did they like what you were wearing? Although there may be signs of social change, traditionally girls are valued for their appearance. If they look nice, they are loved. Unfortunately, this suggests that if they don't look so nice, they are not loved, and maybe they're unlovable.

The message that girls are lovable only when they look good comes at you from all sides. When you went to school, the primers used to teach you to read showed that girls were usually concerned about their looks, but boys never were. The boys were playing games or pretending to do work like their dads. The girls in the readers busied themselves with social activities or dressed up to look like their moms. When you came home from school and turned on the television, the stories were more complex than Dick and Jane, but the same themes were there: Men did all sorts of useful things, but women were lovable only when they were thin and beautiful. Girls still learn this lesson well. Studies have shown that, even in grade school, weight is critical for girls' self-esteem. The thinner girls felt that they were popular, more attractive, and better students than their plumper peers. Boys were just as unhappy if they were underweight as when they were overweight, but girls were dissatisfied only when they were overweight.[6]

Puberty, Love, and Diet

So unconscious patterns of using food to soothe feelings of loneliness were established in your infancy. By middle childhood, your culture, including your parents, have taught you that you must be thin to be lovable. As you enter adolescence, your body is going to make some amazing changes that will impact your eating. Without any effort on your part, you will gain body fat in all sorts of interesting places. Before puberty, girls have slightly more fat than boys. After puberty, girls with their new curves have almost twice the body fat of their male classmates.[7] This is scary! The teen magazines and all your friends let you know that you need to be thin to be pretty, but you're getting fatter. To add to the confusion, you're going to encounter the pressures of dating and sexuality. If it hasn't already happened, soon boys will be asking you out on dates and you'll have to deal with their ever more insistent demands for sex. What do you do now? Your feelings are confused; it's hard to put them into words. Talking about boys and sex with your parents is risky (or maybe impossible), your girlfriends don't know any more than you do, so you deal with the confusion by going on a diet. If you can control your eating, you should be able to discipline your body and bring some order to your chaotic adolescent life. For many women, this is the start of a lifelong pattern of using diets to cope with the confused feelings about men and sexuality.

Cheryl, a 16-year-old high school junior, was in a panic

about her weight. At our first session, Cheryl told me twice, "It would be the end of the world if I put on more weight." She currently weighed 136, but she had gained 11 pounds in the past few weeks. She was afraid that she would quickly get back to the 165 pounds she weighed when she met Eric.

Eric was Cheryl's first love. They met at a pizza parlor and went out for nine months. She adored Eric. Despite her conservative upbringing, she gave in and had sex with him several weeks after they started dating. In her mind, this meant that they would get married. Eric did not share her commitment. Throughout their relationship, Eric had reservations. Unfortunately, he wasn't able to discuss them with Cheryl. Instead he focused on her body, frequently making negative comments about her weight or what she ate. For example, he told her that going to the prom with her was embarrassing because his friends made nasty comments about her figure. To try to win Eric's love, Cheryl gave up her favorite foods (no more pizza, chips, candy bars, or any desserts) and started running every day. It didn't work. Even at 125 pounds, she still wasn't good enough and Eric eventually ended the relationship.

In our sessions Cheryl was totally preoccupied with her diet and weight. Eating (or not eating) and weighing were tangible. If I had let her, she would have talked endlessly about her diets and what she ate. She felt that she should be able to control her eating, and eventually win Eric back. On the other hand, her feelings of rejection, hurt, and humiliation were more confusing, harder to talk about, and seemed impossible to control. So she put all her energy into resisting the pizza her friends were eating and checking the results on the scale. The connection between food and love that started in infancy, and developed in childhood, emerged in her relationships with men and in her feelings about sexuality. As long as Cheryl was preoccupied with her weight and ignoring her emotions, stable weight control was impossible and developing a satisfactory relationship was unlikely. When she finally confronted the hurt, and started to understand her attraction to Eric despite his consistent lack of interest in her, the preoccupation with food and weight decreased. She gained a few pounds and then her weight stabilized.

Think about your own experience. When you were dating and there was conflict, or if you've ever thought seriously about divorce, did you become more preoccupied with your diet? Did losing weight take on a new sense of urgency? Did you feel that things would improve, or you'd be able to cope better when you reached your target weight?

Disconnecting Food from Love

In order to lose weight permanently, it is necessary to disconnect food from love. The bad news is that you can't go back and relive your infancy, childhood, and adolescence to undo the food-love connection. The good news is that you don't have to. You can learn to accept food for what it is: a necessary and frequently pleasurable part of your life, but not a substitute for love.

Many women I have worked with have been able to get their husbands' support in disconnecting food from love, and his help in changing eating patterns. A review of 13 different studies shows that there is greater weight loss when husbands participate in a program than when wives try to do it on their own.[8] If you can get your husband's support, weight loss will be easier. Even if your husband is skeptical, or doesn't want to get involved, understanding how food became connected to love in your past, and how your marriage continues to affect your weight, can help to disconnect eating from your feelings. When this is accomplished, the battle over your weight will subside, and you can call a truce with your scale. Still, I don't want to give you the impression when you disconnect food from love you will miraculously wake up one morning at your ideal weight. Almost always, weight gain has several causes. You will still need to make changes in your eating and exercise patterns. In the next chapter we'll review seven of the most common reasons for putting on weight so that you can get a better understanding of your unique patterns. This will help you know what is important for you and where to focus your efforts. Let's get started.

CHAPTER 2

Seven Reasons Why I Gained Weight

Are you confused about the cause of weight gain? It seems as if there's a new theory each month. Diets high in fat are responsible for obesity. Or was it carbohydrates? Should I eat rice, or maybe grapefruit? Have you read an article that says that diets don't work, your weight is inherited? If you are tired and perplexed, don't despair. You can stop your search for *the* cause of obesity right here. *There isn't a single reason for obesity; there are many.* Even for one person, you, for example, there are several interacting factors that produce that extra weight. Although there is no way of figuring out exactly the mixture of variables that have created your weight, there are clues that will help you to learn which of the possible reasons is the most important for you. When you have a pretty good idea, then you can start making the changes that will bring you to your new weight.

Reason 1: It's All Your Parents' Fault

Have you read about the discovery of the obesity gene? If you did, were you discouraged because there's nothing you can do about a gene that you inherited? Or were you perhaps a little relieved. After all, if weight is programmed by a gene you inherit, there's nothing you can do about it, so why bother dieting? I hate being a spoilsport, but the news about the obesity gene is not a cause for either despair or relief. Let's look at the actual findings first, then we can draw practical implications for you.

According to recent research, the culprits are a defective gene (the "ob gene"), and leptin, its hormonal messenger. Although the research used mice, the researchers at Rockefeller University in New York believe that the ob gene in humans is similar and works in the same way. Mice with a defect in their ob gene produce less leptin. The scientists think that the leptin circulates in the blood and signals the hypothalamus (part of the brain that regulates basic body processes) to stop eating. Since there is less leptin produced by the defective ob gene, the mice eat more food before they "feel full." As a result, they become obese. In the experiment, obese mice were given daily injections of leptin for two weeks. The mice lost 30 percent of their body weight, all of the loss coming from fat. The loss wasn't magical though. After the injection the mice ate less and exercised more. Four days after starting the injections of leptin, the mice were eating 60 percent less food and were running around their cages more.[9]

Before you run down to the drugstore looking for leptin, you should know that there isn't any human leptin for sale yet. When a safe drug, without significant side effects, does become available (probably in 5–10 years) the results for humans will be less dramatic. Even if a leptin pill made you feel full, most of the other reasons for overeating would be left untreated. Certainly the results for humans would be less dramatic than the results for mice. Mice don't usually eat because it's Thanksgiving, or they smelled cookies baking at the cookie stand in the mall, or because they're feeling sad and lonely. Mice eat because of physical hunger. Your eating is different; you eat when you are not physically hungry.

The importance of nongenetic factors is demonstrated by the results of a recent study by the National Center for Health Statistics. The study shows that the percentage of overweight folks (defined as 20 percent or more above a person's desirable weight) remained steady at 25 percent of the population during the years from 1960 through 1980, but between 1980 and 1991 when the survey was done, the percentage increased to 34 percent.[10] Since evolution proceeds over the course of millions of years, something other than genetics is responsible for the increase in the number of overweight Americans.

One scientist, after reviewing many large-scale studies, concluded that the genetic contribution accounts for between 25 to 40 percent of obesity.[11] It's likely that most excess weight is the result of nongenetic, primarily psychological factors. When a drug becomes available which will make you feel full with less food it should be a great help, but it's unlikely to be the complete solution.

Box 2. A Brief History of the Search for a Cure

In the 1960s amphetamines like dexamphetamine and metamphetamine were widely used for weight control. Although they temporarily suppressed appetite, their effectiveness wore off after several weeks and patients usually regained any weight they had lost. Since they could be addictive, the FDA restricted their use and many states prohibited them completely. In

1992 physicians combined fenfluramine and phentermine ("fen-phen"), two older drugs, to treat obesity. In 1996 the FDA approved Redux (dexfenfluramine) for the treatment of obesity and 18 million prescriptions were written that year. A review of research published in the *Journal of the American Medical Association* concluded that medication, "when combined with appropriate behavioral approaches to change diet and physical activity, helps some obese patients lose weight . . ."[12] Nonetheless in 1997 the FDA asked the manufacturers to withdraw Redux and fenfluramine after reports of heart defects associated with their use. Currently there are several fat-fighting drugs being researched, and a few are likely to be approved. It is also likely that, even if they are safe and there are no side effects, changes in eating and exercise habits will still be necessary for permanent weight control.

Before we look at the other causes of obesity, let's get a rough idea of the role of genetics in your weight gain. At present, there isn't any way of knowing how much of your weight is determined by heredity, but you can get some idea by answering the following questions:

- Have you always been heavy? If you're not sure, look at pictures of you when you were a young child. Do you look overweight in all your childhood pictures? Do you remember comments or being teased about your weight throughout your childhood?
- Is one or both of your parents heavy? Have they been heavy all their life? Are your grandparents, aunts, and uncles heavy also?
- Have there been times in your life when you weren't heavy? Could you maintain a lower weight comfortably for months or years?

If you answered yes to the first two questions and no to the third, it is likely that some aspects of your weight gain are inherited. Perhaps you have inherited a lower Resting Metabolic Rate (the amount of energy your body uses up just to stay alive), or a tendency to be less physically active, or maybe you've inherited a tendency to eat foods high in fats and carbohydrates. Any of these tendencies would make it more difficult to lose weight, but it is unlikely that it would be the sole cause for your weight gain. If you think that your weight has a genetic component, you will need to be realistic in your weight loss goals (see Chapter 6), but don't despair. One study of 600 men and women who had lost an average of 66 pounds and kept it off for more than five years found that more than one quarter of these successful losers had two parents who were overweight.[13] These findings suggest that, despite any genetic limitations, you will be able to make significant progress on several of the other factors, and lose weight.

Reason 2: You're Slowing Down

Are you heavier now than when you were 18? For both men and women, the average weight increases until middle age, and then starts to decline in old age. Typically a man's weight increases until age 60, while women keep gaining until they reach 70.[14] The weight gain is probably due to a combination of physiological and lifestyle changes.

The most important change is the decrease in physical activity that is common in adulthood. Compared with high school, when you took gym and may have played sports, it's likely that you get less exercise now. Look at the list of activities on page 42. Put a check in the first column if you routinely and consistently do the activity now, and a check in the second column if you routinely did it when you were a teenager or young adult.

Activity	Now	Teen or Young Adult
Ride a bicycle		
Play sports (once a week or more)		
Aerobic dance		
Swimming		
Exercise program (gym, stationary bicycle)		
Skiing		
Jog, run, or brisk walk		

Do you see any differences? What may be less obvious, but equally important, is a decrease in physical activities that are part of your daily routines. Using the list below, compare your current activity level with your activity when you were younger.

Activity	Now	Teen or Young Adult
Walk to school (or work, shopping, visiting friends)		
Work on your feet (e.g., waitress, salesperson)		
Get up to change TV channels		
Walk up stairs		
Frequent sex		
Wash your car by hand		
Mow lawn, garden		
Open garage door manually		

These lists should give you a few ideas about changes in your activity level. Can you think of other changes that I left out of the lists? Give it a little thought, then write down physical activities or routines that you're not doing anymore:

1. _____   4. _____

2. _____   5. _____

3. _____   6. _____

Eileen, a 28-year-old mother of two, and part-time manager of an apartment complex, is a good example. Although the primary reason she consulted me was because of her obsessive-compulsive rituals (frequent hand washing and constant checking and re-checking of doors, windows, etc.), she also expressed concern about her weight. She wasn't overweight as a child and her parents were not heavy, so there was no evidence of an inherited predisposition to gain weight. When I asked about her activity level, it was clear that there have been major changes.

Eileen described herself as a "tomboy" when she was a kid. She loved to play baseball with her brothers. In high school she was a cheerleader, played volleyball, was on the swimming team, and went to all the high school dances. Within a year after graduating from high school, she married Bill, who had just started working for the state highway department. They had two boys and she got a job managing the apartment complex they lived in so that she could spend more time with her children.

Although chasing after two young children burned up a few calories, in a few years' time, Eileen had made the transition from an active life to a sedentary one. She had given up virtually all of her sports—now when she went into the pool it was to watch her kids, not to race or swim laps. She and Bill rarely went dancing anymore. They bought a television with a remote and an upright vacuum cleaner that propelled itself when you touched the handle. Although her energy expenditure (exercise) dropped dramatically, her energy intake (eating) stayed the same as when she was younger. She had gained more than 40 pounds since high school.

Everyone knows that physical activity uses energy (calories) that otherwise would have become fat tissue. The more you exercise, the more calories you use. This is the direct benefit of physical activity. What is less well known is that there are at least two other physical processes that occur in the body that indirectly help to keep weight down. These are the "fringe benefits" of an active lifestyle.

The first fringe benefit is the increase in metabolic rate that occurs while you exercise, and continues for some time after you have finished. In addition to the calories used in the activity, the number of calories you use for breathing, pumping blood throughout your body, and other routine bodily functions increases, and this increase continues even after you have stopped exercising.

The second fringe benefit is that muscle tissue is more expensive than fat tissue. It costs more calories (not dollars) to maintain an ounce of muscle than an ounce of fat. This means that when you are just sitting there, daydreaming or watching the tube, your muscle tissue is burning up more calories than the same amount of fat tissue is burning, even though neither is doing anything. One estimate is that muscle is about 60 percent more active than fat.[15] So when you exercise, you increase muscle tissue, which continues to use more calories indefinitely.

When Eileen was younger and more physically active, a greater proportion of her body consisted of muscle. As she gave up her activities, she lost muscle tissue and gained weight. Although it may seem natural to gain weight with age, it may be possible to prevent at least some of the usual weight gain with age by maintaining or increasing the muscles you had when you were younger.

The change from an active to a sedentary lifestyle takes place slowly and with it comes the triple whammy that puts on the pounds. Even if the thought of *exercise* has all the appeal of a root canal, in Chapter 12 you'll see how you and your husband can overcome the psychological barriers to increased activity. You will develop an active lifestyle without pain and suffering. You can grow older without growing heavier!

Reason 3: You Are What You Eat

Okay, it's time to look at the most obvious causes of weight gain, what you eat and how much you eat of it. Most diet plans discuss foods and portions together but this is confusing if you are going to understand how you gained weight. Instead, look at food choices (Reason 3) first, and then we can consider food quantity (Reason 4).

Until recently the conventional wisdom was a calorie is a calorie; you gained weight because you consumed more calories than you needed. Lately you've heard that calories don't count; fat grams do. You gained weight when your diet was more than 30 percent fat. Confused? There's some truth in both views.

The typical American diet is high in both grams of fat and calories. According to one estimate, 32 percent of the American diet in 1910 was composed of fat, but by 1989 it had increased to 43 percent.[16] Whether you are counting calories or fat grams, a high-fat diet is bad news. If you are counting calories, fat provides 252 calories per ounce, which is more than twice as many calories per ounce as protein or carbohydrates.

Food with a high-fat content produces weight gain more easily than less fatty foods with an equal number of calories.

It's as though the fat in foods has a head start in the race to become flab on your thighs. When you eat fatty foods, the weight gain is quicker because it takes about 25 percent less energy for the fat in the food to become the fat on your body. This principle was succinctly stated by Dr. John McDougall, a guru of the low-fat movement, "The fat you eat is the fat you wear."

The effects of the typical high-fat American diet were demonstrated in a recent study that compared Japanese-American men with a comparable group of Japanese men who lived in Japan and ate the traditional rice-based Japanese diet. The Japanese-American men were more than two times as likely to become obese.[17]

Box 3. On the Side

When you go to a restaurant, do you ask to have sauce or dressing "on the side"? If you're not careful, you may end up with more fat rather than less. According to one chef, he usually puts an ounce of sauce on a piece of fish, but when he puts the sauce in a server "on the side," a single ounce looks too skimpy. To make it look better, he puts four ounces of sauce in the server. Guess what? Those fat-conscious dieters usually use all four ounces.[18] Although they are trying to be conscientious, they ended up eating more fat. If you order your sauce or dressing on the side, be very careful and only use a little. For example, instead of pouring dressing on your salad, try dipping your fork in the dressing, and then taking a bite of the salad.

If everything else stays the same and you reduce the fat in your diet, you should lose weight. Unfortunately, everything else doesn't always stay the same.

Reason 4: Bigger Is Not Better

Even on a low-fat diet, you can gain weight the good old-fashioned way: consuming too many calories. The easiest way to do this is just to eat too much food. Even if you are conscientious and read the nutrition labeling on food packages, you may be eating more than you think. For example, most labels on pasta provide the caloric value for an uncooked two-ounce serving, but no one eats two ounces of pasta. Most cookbooks recommend four ounces, and in restaurants the serving may be seven or eight ounces. So, when you sit down to your low-fat spaghetti dinner, you are consuming at least 400 calories instead of the 200 on the label. Then you add the sauce, parmesan cheese, garlic bread . . .

It's even worse if you eat out. A 3-ounce baked potato weighs in at a reasonable 120 calories. Yet one Chicago steakhouse routinely serves 1-pound potatoes (that's over 600 calories). The nouvelle cuisine of the 1980s, a small portion of food on a large plate, is a thing of the past. Now the same large plate is covered with food. According to the owner of several upscale New York restaurants, "Our average portion of fish is 13 ounces . . . restaurants serving minute portions have gone out of business."[18] With more Americans eating out more often, weights are increasing despite the emphasis on low-fat foods.

Box 4. The See Food Diet

When there is food on the plate in front of you, what do you do? You eat. This is the see food diet: when you see food, you eat it. Here are a few tips to help you see less food:

1. When you eat at home, don't serve family style. Instead of having the food on the table where you have

to look at it, serve the food in the kitchen and bring the plates to the table. If you really are hungry and need more food, you can always go back into the kitchen for seconds.

2. Store all the food in the house in the refrigerator and kitchen cabinets or pantry. Make sure there are no snacks on the coffee table in the living room, no treats in your dresser drawers, or munchies in the glove box in your car.

3. If you must have high-fat, high-calorie snacks in the house, buy them in single-serving packages even if it is more expensive. With a half gallon of ice cream (or even with a half gallon of nonfat yogurt), it is not easy to regulate your portion. You know that you're having a bowl of ice cream, but how big is the bowl, and are you going to sample a little directly from the container? Instead of dealing with this temptation, buy packaged frozen yogurt cups. When you take one out of the freezer, you know that this is your portion.

4. When you are going to a favorite restaurant with your husband or a friend, consider ordering one full meal, an additional salad, and an extra plate. You can each have your own salad and can split the entrée.

5. When you're at a restaurant and the servings are large, ask for the "doggie bag" as soon as they bring the food. Before you start to eat, divide the foods into the portion that you will eat and the portion that you will take home. As soon as the waitperson returns with the container, put the food that you are going to take home into the container and place the container out of view.

Reason 5: It's All Around You

Even if you've been on a diet during the month of November, it's unlikely that you'll have pasta salad as your dinner on Thanksgiving. Eating doesn't occur in a vacuum. Your eating habits are not just a matter of reading the nutrition labels and making food choices. The environment around you including your family, social groups, and culture all influence your eating. When you're in a foreign country, it's easy to see how culture influences eating patterns and food choices. The English stop everything for afternoon tea (frequently accompanied by biscuits or little sandwiches). In some cultures insects are a delicacy and cow's milk is seen as a disgusting liquid. It's not always obvious, but when we look at our own culture, we can find rituals which have contributed to your weight gain.

Like Thanksgiving, most celebrations are associated with overeating. Having seconds (or thirds or fourths) of each of the wide variety of foods is almost required. If you resist, it's likely that you'll be pressured to comply. In addition to Thanksgiving, add Christmas and Easter dinners, birthday parties, weddings and bar mitzvahs, office parties, and family dinners. Depending on how busy your social calendar is, you may have several meals each month in which you are presented with a large number of attractive high-fat, high-calorie foods.

Some rituals are more subtle. In many workplaces, at 10:30 each morning everything stops for a coffee break. It isn't mandatory that you drink coffee and eat doughnuts, but often this is the expectation. If you decided that you weren't going to drink coffee and eat, but rather spend 10 minutes reading a magazine, would you feel funny? There might be social pressure to join in. You would need to at least appear to be eating something in order to fit in. If you review your own eating, you may find other social rituals that seem to require eating. Are you expected to snack when your husband is watching football? Do the members of your bridge group try to outdo each other serving fancy desserts?

Starting in childhood with birthday cakes and Halloween candy, progressing to the parties and rituals of adulthood, your social environment has added pounds and interfered with your attempts to diet.

Reason 6: Seeking Comfort in Food

In Chapter 1, I briefly discussed the effects of emotions on eating. To estimate how significant this is for you, look at the list of feelings below. Think about each, and as honestly as possible, indicate the extent to which the feeling leads to an urge to eat. Put a check in the appropriate box.

	No Desire to Eat	A Small Desire to Eat	A Moderate Desire to Eat	A Strong Urge to Eat	An Overwhelming Urge to Eat
Resentful					
Discouraged					
Shaky					
Worn-out					
Inadequate					
Excited					
Rebellious					
Blue					
Jittery					
Sad					
Uneasy					
Irritated					

	No Desire to Eat	A Small Desire to Eat	A Moderate Desire to Eat	A Strong Urge to Eat	An Overwhelming Urge to Eat
Jealous					
Worried					
Frustrated					
Lonely					
Furious					
On edge					
Confused					
Nervous					
Angry					
Guilty					
Bored					
Helpless					
Upset					

You have just completed the Emotional Eating Scale developed by Dr. Bruce Arnow and his colleagues at the Stanford University Medical School.[19] Your scores on this scale will help identify any relationships between negative emotions and eating. To score the scale, look at the three lists of feelings. In the space next to each feeling, give yourself one point if you checked "No desire to eat," a two if you checked "A small desire to eat," a three for "A moderate desire to eat," a four for "A strong urge to eat," and five for "An overwhelming urge to eat."

_____ Discouraged	_____ Helpless
_____ Guilty	_____ Resentful
_____ Irritated	_____ Frustrated

_____ Angry	_____ Jealous
_____ Furious	_____ Rebellious
_____ Inadequate	_____ *Total*

_____ Jittery	_____ Uneasy
_____ On edge	_____ Worried
_____ Shaky	_____ Upset
_____ Nervous	_____ Confused
_____ Excited	_____ *Total*

_____ Lonely	_____ Blue
_____ Bored	_____ Worn-out
_____ Sad	_____ *Total*

For each of the three groups of feelings, add up your points and put the result in the space labeled "Total." The first group of feelings measures anger and frustration, the second group is anxiety, and the third is depression. To help you make sense of your scores, compare your totals with a group of overweight women who started a treatment program for binge eating and weight loss, and with another group without eating problems.

	Overweight Patients	Normal-Weight Patients
Anger and frustration	25.4	5.1
Anxiety	15.9	4.0
Depression	12.5	5.2

How do your scores compare? Are they similar to the group of overweight patients? If so, it is likely that emotional eating plays a significant role in your weight gain, and will need to be controlled for you to make progress losing weight.

Many dieters report that they have had some success

controlling what they eat until they are emotionally upset. Following an emotional disturbance, they give up on their diet, but they don't resume "normal" eating; they go on an eating binge. This is the most destructive pattern of emotional eating, but not the only one. In my earlier book, *Emotional Eating: What You Need to Know Before Starting Another Diet* (Jossey-Bass Publishers, 1998), I described in detail different patterns of emotional eating and their relationship to gaining weight.

In addition to contributing to weight gain, emotional eating may be responsible for your previous difficulties sticking to a diet. One study of dieters in a hospital-based program found that almost half of the time dieters gave up, it was following an unpleasant emotion.[20] In an English study dieters took a scale similar to the Emotional Eating Scale you just completed before they began a weight loss program. They took the same scale a year later. The researchers found that dieters who were able to curb their emotional eating lost more weight than dieters who didn't.[21] If you had high scores on any of the three Emotional Eating Scales, coping with anger/frustration, depression, and anxiety without eating will be essential to make any weight loss program successful. You will learn how to do this in Chapters 7 and 9.

Reason 7: Pregnancy and Life Changes

Many women attribute their weight gain to pregnancy, but it usually isn't that straightforward. Biologically, it is useful for a normal weight woman to gain between 25 to 35 pounds during pregnancy (although women who are overweight should gain less[22]). The extra weight is necessary for nursing since mothers only eat enough to provide 60 percent of the energy that their baby needs. Research shows that, despite the weight gain during pregnancy, the average mother is only 3 pounds heavier after the child is born.[23] If a mother-to-be doesn't breastfeed her baby, she'll keep more of the weight she gained while pregnant (an extra 6 pounds, according to one recent study[24]). Although the biology of pregnancy may add only a few pounds, becoming a mother starts a sequence that makes losing weight difficult. A study in Sweden found that lifestyle change during and after pregnancy was the most important cause of weight retention after childbirth.[25] In Chapter 3 you will identify the lifestyle changes that followed your pregnancy and added pounds. In Part II you will learn to reverse them.

Pregnancy isn't the only change that can add pounds. Looking back, was there a period where you gained a substantial amount of weight in a brief period of time? For example, Jean, a 46-year-old gym teacher, was an active woman who, despite her large frame, had always been able to maintain her weight by a combination of physical activity and minimizing the fat in her diet. About three years before our first session she injured her knee and had to give up running. At about the same time, her stormy relationship with her husband got worse. One side effect was her nightly glass of wine with dinner increased to several glasses and mixed drinks later in the evening. Since her knee injury Jean gained more than 25 pounds.

Jean's example shows how a change can produce a weight gain. As she described the period following the injury, it became apparent that she had become mildly depressed when she had to give up her exercise routine. Her depression produced more conflict with her husband and more drinking. By the time she came to see me, she had given up exercising, was drinking excessively (alcohol doesn't have any fat, but is high in calories), and was using food and alcohol to deal with her emotional turmoil.

Although her weight gain had several causes, the knee injury started the process.

If you think about your own weight gain, you may be able to identify a change that started the process. As in Jean's case, it may have been an injury or illness, but it also could have been the loss of a job, moving to a new town, or even a lengthy vacation. This one change didn't produce the weight gain by itself but it may have started a sequence that eventually resulted in weight gain.

Another change that could add weight is quitting smoking. Several studies indicate that average weight gains of 10 pounds are quite common but 15 to 20 percent of ex-smokers could gain 30 pounds or more.[26] If you have given up smoking, give yourself a pat on the back, even if you've gained weight. The health risks associated with smoking are much worse than those with weight gain. You'd have to be at least 100 to 150 pounds overweight before you have the health problems of a smoker.[27]

If you are a recent quitter and are gaining weight, or if you'd like to quit but are afraid that you would gain, you might want to try nicotine gum. Research shows that, at the very least, the gum will postpone weight gain[28] so you don't have to tackle two major changes at the same time. After you are comfortable without cigarettes, you can work on losing weight.

Finding Your Profile

Have you come to any conclusions about your weight gain? Most participants in my workshops can identify with several of the seven reasons. Briefly review the seven reasons, and make a check for each to indicate how important it is for you.

Reasons for Weight Gain	Definitely Applies to Me	Might Apply to Me	Definitely Does Not Apply to Me
1. Heredity			
2. Lack of physical activity			
3. High-fat, high-calorie foods			
4. Quantity of food			
5. Culture and rituals			
6. Emotional eating			
7. Pregnancy and life changes			

Many dieters in commercial weight loss programs become frustrated when they find themselves working on problems they don't have. As we proceed, keep in mind which of the reasons for weight gain are most important for you. While you should learn about all of the methods, you can put your energy into the methods that apply to you.

Like you, men and single women become overweight from some combination of the seven reasons but you have an additional reason for gaining: You are a married woman. In Chapter 3 you will see how your marriage could have made you fat. Then we can reverse the process and use your marriage to achieve permanent weight control.

CHAPTER 3

The Eighth Reason: I Got Married

Has your weight changed since you've been married? If you're not sure, find one of your wedding pictures and see how you looked on your wedding day. Do you like what you see? Most women, even those who thought they were overweight at the time, would be thrilled to return to their weight on the day they got married. What happened? Obviously you're older now, so you are probably less active and need less food to keep going (see Reason 2 in Chapter 2), so some of your weight gain comes with age. If you have kids, you might have kept a few pounds after giving birth (see Reason 7). So while age and pregnancy may have contributed to your weight gain, it's likely that something else has been going on. For most women, the lifestyle changes that come with marriage and motherhood are the Eighth Reason.

Lifestyle Changes

To start, think for a minute about how your life has changed from your single days. To help identify a few of these differences, look at the list below. For each statement, put a check in the first column if it describes you when you were single, and a check in the second column if it describes you now.

	When I Was Single	Now That I'm Married
1. I feel that people won't like me if I am overweight.		
2. I eat because I am bored.		
3. I have a full dinner with several courses and dessert.		
4. Other people encourage me to eat what they are eating.		
5. Sometimes I eat to prove a point to someone else.		
6. I need to keep my figure to be sexy.		
7. Snacking provides a break in my routine.		
8. I buy a food because someone else wants it, but then I eat some.		
9. Other people frequently comment about what I am eating or my weight.		
10. Sometimes I eat just to show that no one can tell me what to do.		

	When I Was Single	Now That I'm Married
11. I'm not comfortable socializing if I am overweight.		
12. Usually there is food nearby when I am working.		
13. I keep snack food and desserts in the house.		
14. My diets or weight are discussed when there is a disagreement.		
15. I eat when I am angry with someone else.		

What do you find when you compare your responses in Column 2 to those in Column 1? Do you see any differences? When I gave a similar questionnaire to a group of married women in a workshop I was conducting, everyone could identify several changes since they got married. One woman recalled that, when she was single, she never kept cookies or pastries in her apartment. Another chuckled as she described "the good old days" when she and a roommate would try to eat only vegetables for dinner. They were both dieting, and usually disagreed about whether the main course was going to be squash or broccoli. All of the workshop participants agreed that, after being married for several years, they no longer had the same motivation to diet. Being slim was still desirable, they'd love to lose the weight, but it just didn't have the same sense of urgency that it had before. Why? Of all the changes that come with marriage, the most important is that *you stop dating*.

The Dating Game

Think of dating as a giant, long-term board game. In a board game, you roll the dice and move your token until you reach the finish line. In the Dating Game, instead of moving your token on the board, each time you roll the dice, you land on a square inhabited by another male. Sometimes you land on a square that requires that you give up three rolls of the dice—this is a long-term relationship. More often, after a brief stay (one or two dates), you can't wait until it's your turn so that you can roll the dice again. Occasionally, you land on a square that makes you move back four spaces and skip a turn. You are dating your old boyfriend for a while, but then you pick up the dice and try your luck again. The Dating Game continues until you land on the square with Mr. Right. You fall in love, and get married. The game is over, you've won.

In a board game all you have to do is flick your wrist to toss the dice. In the Dating Game, rolling the dice takes more effort. Actually, it requires that you watch your weight by planning your meals, giving up foods that you enjoy, feeling hungry some of the time, deprived most of the time, and doing exercises that leave you sweaty and out-of-breath. You do this for years until you win the Dating Game, but what do you do when the game is over? If you win a board game, do you continue to roll the dice? Of course not, it's pointless. For the Dating Game it makes even less sense. Dieting is hard work, you've already won, so why bother?

Look at your responses to the Single-Married Checklist. Pay particular attention to numbers 1, 6, and 11. Has your attitude toward dieting changed since you've been married? Now that the Dating Game is over, there is less motivation to deprive yourself. With all the time-consuming demands of marriage, watching your weight moved lower on your list of priorities. It becomes something you *should* do as soon as (choose one): you have more time, you're less stressed at work, the kids are older, or you can afford to join a fitness club. If this sounds familiar, and you're starting to feel a little guilty, you can relax and go easy on yourself. The reality is that as long as you stay married (and even if you don't stay married), your motivation to diet will never be as great as it was when you were younger, single, and playing the Dating Game. The good news is that losing weight doesn't require the same sense of urgency and restraint that you remember from your single days. Instead of a desperate crash diet so you can look good for your date next Friday, you will develop a more relaxed, but consistent plan for weight control so you can look and feel good for the rest of your life.

Life After the Dating Game

Now that you've won the Dating Game and have settled into married life, it is time to assume your wifely duties. Even in the most egalitarian marriages, even when your husband really is thoughtful and tries to help, the primary responsibility for shopping, food preparation, serving, and cleaning up is still yours. For most women, this is a major change from single life when you shared these tasks with your mother, a dormitory cook, or a roommate. Even if you lived alone when you were single, you only had the responsibility for feeding yourself. You did not have the added demands of feeding a husband and children.

Box 5. Dodging Land Mines in the Supermarket Battlefield

When was the last time you bought something really good, brought it home, decided that it was fattening, and threw it away without eating any? Not recently, I'll bet. When you buy something you like, you're going to eat it unless someone else gets there first. To decrease the fattening foods in your diet, you'll need to avoid them in the supermarket so you aren't faced with continued temptation at home. While you may need to buy some fattening foods for other family members (see Chapter 11), you still can cut back on your purchases of fattening foods. Using these strategies will help you navigate the minefield in the supermarket.

1. Never shop on an empty stomach. When you're hungry, everything looks good.

2. Prepare a shopping list at home and stick to it in the supermarket.

3. If you're just running in to grab something from the dairy case (almost always located in the back of the store), walk through the side aisles rather than through the center of the store. The side aisles usually have meat or fruits and vegetables. You're not likely to grab a head of lettuce because it looks good.

4. If you are doing your major shopping, listen to a Walkman in the store. This will help you avoid thinking about the foods that you are passing by and keep your focus on the foods on your list.

5. When you are ready to check out, choose a lane that doesn't have candy displays to tempt you. If all the cash registers are surrounded by racks of candy bars, pick up a supermarket tabloid, and become engrossed in the story of the latest Elvis sighting until it is your turn at the cash register.

Married life becomes more fattening when you have children. You have to patiently feed infants and toddlers, get milk and cookies for returning elementary school kids, have frozen pizzas available at all hours for teenagers, and deal with all the leftovers. If you are a full-time, stay-at-home mom with one or more little ones, you are never more than a few feet from the refrigerator or a few minutes from a demand for food. Marriage counselors Richard Stuart and Barbara Jacobson call full-time motherhood, "the most fattening job in the world."[29] A stay-at-home mom spends her whole workday a few feet away from the refrigerator. Even if she tried to forget all the goodies nearby, one of her major job responsibilities—planning and preparing meals—would remind her. Her routine combines easy access to food with a variety of boring tasks and a lack of adult daytime companionship. This combination makes having a snack the exciting break in her routine. For the stay-at-home mom, the leftover piece of pie may be the high point of the afternoon. Contrast this with your life as a single person. If you were in school or working, you didn't have continued access to food all day long. Even if you worked in a restaurant, there were restrictions on how much and when you could eat. At home the refrigerator is always beckoning.

Marie, a 32-year-old former teacher who was staying home to raise her two young children, described the role that food played in her afternoons:

Usually I wake up with my husband, feed the kids, take them to preschool, rush to do the food shopping and other chores, pick them up, make lunch, try to spend a little time with them, and then hope that they both take a nap at the same time. Every day, as soon as I drop the kids off at preschool, I am planning my midafternoon snack. I look forward to sitting down, by myself, and having something good to eat. Sometimes thinking about the snack gets the better of me, and I eat it before the kids take a nap. Then I have to find something else to eat when I get my break.

Three years earlier, when Marie was still teaching, there were no midafternoon snacks. Marie has gained almost 20 pounds since she's been at home.

Although he hardly qualifies as a stay-at-home mom, best-selling novelist John Updike (author of *Rabbit, Run* and 16 other novels) also works at home and experiences the same temptations. In a recent interview, he discussed this problem:

> *There's no disguising the fact that a writer's life is a sedentary one and prone to incessant snacking if you work at home. The little break of going down to get another oatmeal cookie is almost irresistible.*[30]

I agree. As I'm writing this (at home), the thought of an oatmeal cookie is very appealing. Fortunately, we don't have any in the house (see Box 5).

Check your responses to numbers 2, 7, and 12 to see if the responsibilities of motherhood and running a household have contributed to your weight gain.

Box 6. Being Bored

Many household chores and work assignments are repetitive and uninteresting. Confronted with a pile of clothes to be ironed, it is difficult to become totally involved with the task at hand. If you are bored at home, sooner or later the thought will pop into your head, "I wonder what goodies there are in the refrigerator." Despite your resolve to finish the task, it's likely that you'll take a break and reward yourself with whatever you find. If you are bored at work, you may also daydream about food, but unless it's time for a coffee break or you have a stash of snacks in your desk drawer, eating is not as easy.

To decrease eating out of boredom, plan to do boring tasks in places where food is hard to get. If you are a student and you are dreading the chapters you need to read in your boring chemistry textbook, plan to do your reading in the library, away from the candy machines. If you can't put off ironing any longer, take the wash, your ironing board, and a portable TV out to the garage and do your ironing there. Most libraries and garages don't have any visible food cues to entice you. It is still possible to snack, but the effort it takes to get food will make it less automatic.

The Declaration of Dietary Dependence

Even if you are not a stay-at-home Mom (or a stay-at-home author), your eating is at least partially controlled by your spouse. When Kristin was 18, she graduated from high school and moved to a nearby city to start her studies to become a legal secretary. During the weekdays, she lived with her sister in an apartment, returning to her hometown on weekends so she could see her boyfriend, Peter. Some weeknights Kristin stopped to pick up a salad on the way home. Other nights she and her sister took turns preparing dinner, often chicken breasts and salad, or a tuna salad. When she married Peter a year later, her eating habits changed dramatically. She gave up control over her meals. In effect, when she signed the marriage license, she put her Jane Hancock on a Declaration of Dietary Dependence.

Peter liked pot roast and mashed potatoes with gravy, or fried chicken and mashed potatoes with gravy, or meat loaf and mashed potatoes with gravy. No meal was complete without a heaping bowl of ice cream, preferably rocky road. After their first child was born, an additional element was added to Kristin's dietary routine: home-baked cakes and cookies. Peter's mom saw rich meals and high-calorie treats as a sign of a loving home. Peter naturally assumed that his new wife would create the same kind of home regardless of her own food preferences. Kristin did not disappoint him. Peter, a physically active contractor, was able to eat all this food and gain only a few pounds. Kristin wasn't as fortunate. She gained 30 pounds in five years of marriage.

It's not unusual for women living together to do their own shopping and cooking. When you were single, if your roommate's favorite dinner was meat loaf with mashed potatoes and gravy, would you feel obligated to provide it for her? It's unlikely that your roommate's appetites and preferences determined what you were going to eat—she could make her own meat loaf. Now that you're married, it's not that simple. Your eating is affected by the preferences of your husband and kids. You've lost your dietary independence.

Can you identify changes in your eating habits that began when you became responsible for the meals of your husband and children? To get a few clues, go back to the Single-Married Checklist and look at numbers 3, 8, and 13. Are you eating fuller meals and buying foods and snacks that your husband and children want? These are just a few examples of the loss of dietary independence.

Keeping up with your husband's eating habits can produce significant weight gain. It may not be fair, but your husband can eat more than you do without gaining weight. According to one rule of thumb, every day men need to consume 12 calories for each pound in order to maintain a stable body weight. Women need only 11 calories to keep their weight constant.[31] While it doesn't sound like much of a difference, over time it adds up. If both you and your husband weigh 150 pounds, are equally active, and consume an identical 1,800 calories per day, you will gain and he won't. Estimating that 3,500 excess calories yields a one-pound weight gain, at the end of a year your husband will still weigh 150 pounds while you will weigh 165. Dietary dependence is fattening.

Box 7. Dining with Your Husband

Just because you are having dinner with your husband doesn't mean that you have to eat everything that he does. While it might feel awkward to sit at the table just watching your husband eat, you can eat for the same amount of time as he does without eating the same amount of food that he does. A few tricks will help:

1. Don't serve "family style." Dish out your food in the kitchen and leave the bowls in the kitchen. Put less food on your plate than you put on his.

2. Eat slowly. While you are chewing, put your knife and fork down. Don't pick them up again until you have swallowed.

3. Toward the middle of the meal, put your knife and fork down for one minute. The food is still yours, no one will take it away, but the pause will help slow the pace of eating.

4. If it looks like you will finish before your husband, leave a small amount of food on your plate, but stop eating.

Dieting with Your Husband

Now let's fast-forward into the future. You've won the Dating Game, got married, lost your dietary independence, and spend at least some time working in the kitchen. You've gained weight, so it's time to go on a diet. You dieted before when you were playing the Dating Game and usually lost a few pounds, so you should be able to do it again. Right? Well, not exactly. Married dieting is different from single dieting. Not only is the sense of urgency that you had when playing the Dating Game gone, but now when you try to lose weight, you are not alone—there is a husband looking over your shoulder and making comments. Since he views dieting from a male perspective, he doesn't understand your experience. His comments are not likely to be helpful.

If you have been overweight for some time, those excess pounds may have become part of a delicate mechanism that maintains the balance in your relationship. Sarah, a 37-year-old mother of two had gained more than 50 pounds during 11 years of marriage. She felt miserable about her weight and had made several serious attempts to diet. Typically, she would lose 20 pounds or more, but always got discouraged and regained the weight. She told me:

> Something is standing in the way of being successful. The closer I get to my goal, the more disturbed I feel. I tried to ask Jerry [her husband] for help, but I didn't want to make it his responsibility.

As we discussed her dieting history, it became clear that Sarah needed help from Jerry in two areas: accepting a few changes in routine, and providing emotional support that would keep her motivated as she changed her eating habits. Unfortunately this help wasn't forthcoming. For example, she asked Jerry if he would take the kids out to get yogurt a couple of nights each week so that they didn't have to keep ice cream in the house. He grudgingly agreed, but sometimes "forgot" and brought a half gallon of ice cream home for dessert. When Sarah came home excited from her weekly meetings with the diet program counselor, she was expecting some praise and enthusiasm from Jerry.

Instead, she got a perfunctory "that's good" followed by a quick change of topic. As her weight decreased, Jerry's critical comments increased. Sarah was confused:

> *He became more concerned about what I was eating. Anytime I started to eat something that wasn't on my diet, he would make a nasty comment about how I should stick to my diet. Other times when I passed up a tempting food, he tried to convince me that it was okay for me to try some. He also started complaining about the cost of my diet program, and acted hurt when I went out to walk with my friend Jennifer. He's always wanted me to lose weight, but he doesn't seem very happy when I did lose.*

The Diet Equilibrium

Sarah didn't know why she was getting mixed messages from Jerry. As is usually the case, the use of weight and diets to maintain the equilibrium in a marriage was a gradual development. In the 11 years they had been married, Jerry used Sarah's increasing weight to win arguments and sometimes to avoid responsibilities. This was not a deliberate plan on his part. When Jerry expressed disappointment about her weight, Sarah felt guilty and usually backed down from making demands of him. As a result, when there was conflict, Jerry fell into the habit of using Sarah's weight to demonstrate that she was wrong. Whatever the validity of her point of view, the discussion would end when Jerry, in an angry or sarcastic tone, reminded her that she had failed at dieting and therefore was untrustworthy, incompetent, or had poor judgment.

On the rare occasions when Sarah was critical of Jerry or made demands of him, he would discount her complaints because she still hadn't lost enough weight. For example,

Sarah described a recent conversation in which she complained to Jerry when he was late coming home:

SARAH: Where have you been? You said you'd be home by eleven and it's twelve-fifteen.

JERRY: I said I'd be home *around* eleven. I started to leave, but I just lost track of the time.

SARAH: What do you mean, you just lost track of the time. You have a watch. At least you could have called so I'd know that you're okay. You're so inconsiderate.

JERRY: All right, I said I'm sorry. I just forgot that's all.

SARAH: Forget? How can you forget for an hour and fifteen minutes?

JERRY: Look, you forget your diet all the time, so give me a break. I didn't give you crap when you *forgot* about having fruit and helped yourself to that chocolate cake your mother made.

Over the years a finely balanced equilibrium had developed in Sarah and Jerry's marriage. Unfortunately, the balance included Sarah's 50-pound weight gain and her guilty feelings about it (see Figure 1). When she started to lose, the balance was upset and Jerry went to great lengths to restore the balance by helping her regain the weight. As we shall see in Chapter 10, there are many techniques husbands use to restore the balance.

Often husbands are not aware of their role in maintaining their wife's weight. Even when other aspects of the relationship are good, weight becomes part of the equilibrium in the marriage. Check your responses to numbers 4, 9, and 14 on the Single-Married Checklist. Does your husband give you mixed messages about your weight and eating? When you argue, does the focus shift to your diet? Chapter 10 will show you how to remove weight from the equilibrium.

Figure 1

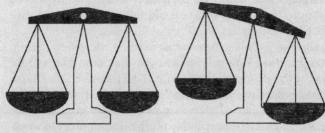

When Sarah is overweight   When Sarah loses weight

The Unhappy Marriage

So far, we've been examining marriages where both partners are reasonably content. Now, let's consider what happens if your marriage has been troubled for some time. Like most married women, you've given up strenuous dieting and taken on weight-producing daily tasks. In addition to the usual reasons for post-marital weight gain, you have an additional reason for gaining weight: you've become resentful. Instead of living happily ever after, you are disappointed, frustrated, and feeling unloved. The hell with the diet, you'll have another piece of pie. A survey of thousands of women responding to a questionnaire in a magazine found that unhappily married women gained an average of over 42 pounds after 13 years of marriage (happily married women still gained 18.4 pounds).[32] Why do unhappily married women gain more weight? Undoubtedly they seek comfort in food (Reason 6 in Chapter 2), but it is likely that something else is happening.

Several women patients have told me that, when their husband was especially frustrating, they ate "to teach him a lesson." This pattern seems most common when he is very controlling. Usually the wife feels that it is pointless to try to disagree with him; it only provokes an argument which she loses. Eventually, she feels misunderstood, frustrated and powerless. The only way she can assert her independence is to eat, preferably foods that he would disapprove of. Rita, a 42-year-old full-time mother of two, is a good example:

Despite Tom's princely charm when they were dating, once married Rita quickly learned that Tom had a rigid view of the proper role of a wife. Tom displayed no charm whatsoever when he felt that Rita strayed from this role. He expected her to take care of their two girls, prepare meals, and take responsibility for the household. On weekends she was to be available to socialize with their friends and to graciously accept his absences when he went hunting or fishing, played basketball, or went bowling. He was not very happy when she went on a shopping expedition with her friends, and absolutely forbade her to take any classes at the local junior college. Most of Rita's attempts to discuss these issues ended when Tom, in an angry tone, said, "It's my way or the highway!" Eventually Rita chose the highway.

When she first came to see me, Rita had been divorced for two years and was enrolled in college. For several difficult years before the divorce, Rita gained weight. As we discussed her marriage during this period, it became clear that much of the weight gain was Rita's way of coping with her anger toward Tom. Eating helped her deal with her anger. Since Tom couldn't monitor every bite she took, it was one way of escaping his control. After a fight, especially when he "laid down the law" to her, Rita found herself snacking. As Rita gained weight, Tom became concerned about the foods she was eating. Sometimes he would tease; other times he would "remind" her to avoid fattening foods. Rita knew that it was silly, but eating junk food became one way of asserting her independence while getting back at Tom.

Look at your responses to numbers 5, 10, and 15 on the Single-Married Checklist. Do you eat to prove a point or to demonstrate that you can't be bossed by your husband? Could your weight gain be a response to being angry and feeling controlled in your marriage? In Chapter 9 you will learn an adaptive way of dealing with your angry feelings so that you won't be tempted to eat.

The Eighth Reason: You Got Married

By now you probably have some ideas about how being married has contributed to your weight gain and interfered with your diets. In Chapter 4 you and your husband will learn to bridge the gender differences so that you can communicate more effectively about weight and diet. Then the two of you will be able to use the methods described in Part II to change habits, lose weight, and improve your relationship.

CHAPTER 4

Lessons in Intergalactic Communication

In Chapter 3 we saw how the changes that come with marriage can add weight. Now we will see how that process can be reversed and your marriage can contribute to weight loss. Actually, even if you are the exception and had most of your weight gain before you got married, having your husband participate would still help you to lose. He can be the secret weapon in your battle for weight control!

Having your husband's help can make the difference between success and another dieting failure. In one study of successful dieters who had maintained their losses for five years or more, nearly 91 percent reported that they had a series of unsuccessful diets, losing and regaining an average of 270 pounds, before they finally succeeded. The single theme that differentiated the successful weight loss from the earlier failures was a greater commitment to making the changes that produced the loss.[33] Now, think about your previous attempts to diet. Remember the days when your commitment faded, when weight loss just didn't seem to be worth the effort. This is when you would give up and start to put the weight back on. Where can you find the commitment that will keep you on your program, even when you're feeling discouraged? You don't have to look any further than the guy you married! Your husband, if he knows what to do, can make the difference (even if he isn't always a prince). Many of the chapters in Part II will include a brief section for your husband to read. It will present straightforward instructions for him to help. If he is hesitant, you can show him why it is to his own benefit to follow these guidelines. If he still refuses to participate, you will learn to proceed when he is not supportive, even if he criticizes your efforts. Hopefully your husband will become an effective support person, but if not, he will lose the ability to undermine the good work you do on your own.

Margaret, a 36-year-old accountant, weighed 165 pounds when she first consulted me. Eight years earlier, she had married Jeff, a short, stocky 44-year-old contractor. Although her weight had remained stable for the first few years of marriage, Margaret had gained almost 30 pounds in the last five years. She attributed most of her weight gain to her two pregnancies. Careful questioning and accurate recording of Margaret's current eating and activity suggested that there had been some weight gain before she became pregnant, and she was currently overeating and underexercising. In addition, there were major changes in her eating habits when she cut her hours at work so she could spend more time at home with her two kids. Although she had tried several diets, and belonged to a commercial weight reduction program for two months, she usually had difficulty maintaining her initial enthusiasm once the novelty wore off. Invariably her commitment decreased, she became discouraged, and she regained any weight she had lost. When we were discussing these dieting failures, she looked ashamed and seemed guilty. She explained her dieting difficulties using vague, negative terms like "lazy" or "no willpower."

When I described how we could involve her husband, Margaret had serious reservations. She gave me a lengthy list of reasons why it would not work:

> *Jeff has been working on a project out-of-town for the last few months so he's only home on weekends. Usually, he comes home tired, so he sleeps in. He spends time with the kids and tries to give me some attention, but there's not much time. I don't see how he could help me lose weight. Besides, he doesn't mind my weight. He's a little overweight himself and gets defensive any time I say anything about it. I really don't think that he would be much help.*

Fortunately I was able to persuade Margaret that it was worth a try. Using some of the materials that are incorporated in this book, she got a halfhearted agreement from Jeff to help. Initially, he did little more than ask, during their nightly phone conversations, how she was doing. Even though Jeff's participation was minimal, his interest and encouragement helped Margaret maintain her commitment after the novelty of a new diet wore off. There were times when her interest waned, but knowing that Jeff was somewhat involved helped Margaret recommit to the plan. As she continued to progress, Jeff became more curious about what she was actually doing to lose weight. Without ever formally announcing that he was going to diet, Jeff started to participate in many of Margaret's weight loss methods. The most obvious change was that they were taking walks together. Jeff also followed Margaret's lead in cutting out fats from his diet and reducing the size of the portions he ate. There was an interesting by-product of these changes: Jeff and Margaret became closer. Between Jeff's out-of-town work and the nonstop demands of raising two small children, they had lost some of the emotional closeness they'd had before the kids were born. Involving Jeff in her weight control program provided a structure for Margaret to take the lead in reestablishing this closeness. The following table shows some of the resulting changes.

Situation	What Jeff Did Before	What Jeff Does Now
Shopping	Brought home forbidden foods. Insisted that we have ice cream and snacks at home.	If he wants high-fat, high-calorie foods, he eats them outside of the house, when I am not with him.
Meals	Offered me seconds when he was having more. Complained if I tried a new low-fat recipe. Nagged if I ate something that wasn't on my diet.	He doesn't try to influence my eating or make comments about what I eat. He tells me his opinion about new recipes, but doesn't complain.
Exercise	Made fun of any attempt I made to exercise. Complained when I went to aerobics class in the evening.	We go on walks together. He accepts that I will spend some time exercising without him.
Socializing	At parties told friends about my dieting failures. Made frequent positive comments about other women's bodies.	He doesn't discuss my diets or weight with other people. He doesn't make comments that might make me feel bad about my body.

I don't want to give you the impression that everything ran smoothly as soon as Margaret consulted me. There were several times when she gave up, feeling that it was futile. Also her first attempts to enlist Jeff's help yielded mixed results. Some days he was pretty negative. Often this produced some conflict with bad feelings lasting several days. A good deal of our sessions were devoted to working through these setbacks.

Although professional help is sometimes necessary, many of the possible detours and dead-ends can be avoided if you can anticipate them in advance and have contingency plans for dealing with them. Each of the chapters in Part II will help you to identify potential pitfalls, and suggest methods for dealing with them.

Women Are from Venus, Men Are from a Different Galaxy

As you read the story of Margaret and Jeff, you may have thought something like, "This is a fairy tale. There's no way my husband would respond like that. Every time the topic of my weight comes up, he either isn't interested and doesn't want to talk, or he makes negative comments and I feel worse than I did before." Although I don't know the details of your marriage, I do know that communication often reaches a stalemate, especially when it revolves around a topic as sensitive as weight.

In his best-selling book, *Men Are from Mars, Women Are from Venus,* marriage counselor John Gray describes gender differences in communication styles. When they are talking about eating and weight, it often seems that men and women are from different galaxies rather than different planets. Men tend to "tune out" their wives when they talk about weight for several reasons. One reason is that your husband thinks that he's heard what you are going to say about your diet or weight dozens of times before so he expects another boring repetition. Another reason for his glazed look when you bring up weight or diet is that he senses that the conversation will end up in an emotionally charged discussion. He's afraid that regardless of what he says, there will be conflict and he will end up feeling bad. To get his help, it will be necessary that Mars and Venus are in the same orbit when they are communicating.

Mars and Venus in the Same Orbit

Since you will be trying to get your husband's help, you'll have to learn his language so that you can ask in terms that will make sense to him. I'm not sure that this is fair—maybe he should learn your language—but since you're the one reading this book, it is the most practical way of solving the communication problem.

Keep in mind that effective communication does *not* mean that you have a perfect marriage with no fights. According to Dr. John Gottman, a psychologist who has studied thousands of couples, a happy marriage can have conflict as long as there are five positive interactions (enjoying a joke together, asking "How was your day?," giving or getting a compliment, or just a simple touch) for each negative interaction (disagreeing, complaining).[34] So if a discussion about your weight or any other topic results in a disagreement, don't get discouraged; just make sure that there are five pleasant events to counteract the disagreement.

Box 8. The Magic 5 to 1 Ratio

Even in the best relationships it doesn't hurt to make a deliberate effort to increase the number of positive interactions you have with your spouse. Think of this as an investment in the future of your relationship. When you have the inevitable conflict, it will be "diluted" in 5 instances of good feelings. The 5 to 1 ratio will keep the relationship strong.

If you think your husband would be receptive, ask him to read this box. It's much easier when both partners are trying to increase good feelings. If he's not interested yet, you can start on your own. Here are a few of Dr. Gottman's suggestions for creating good feelings:

1. Show interest in your husband's activities and hobbies. Ask what he's reading, listen to his stories about his day at work, or discuss politics, sports, or other interests.

2. Be affectionate. This can include sex, but is not limited to making love. If you think he would enjoy it, hold hands at the movies, rub his neck, or just sit closely while you're watching TV together.

3. Be thoughtful. Leave a little note in his car, call in the middle of the afternoon to see how his day is going, or remind him that there was a program he said he wanted to watch. You are letting him know that you think about him.

4. Be playful. Share a joke you think is funny. If you feel comfortable, act silly or do something foolish to make him smile. Teasing can be playful as long as both of you find it fun. Avoid teasing about sensitive topics. Make sure there is no hostility or sarcasm when you joke or tease.

5. Show concern. When you see that your husband is upset (with men it's often expressed as generalized anger or irritability), let him know that you are concerned. Even if you don't agree with his view, show him that you are unhappy when he is upset.

Share your joy. If you are feeling good about something, include your husband. Pay attention to how he responds so that you don't seem to be gloating when he is having a bad day. Let him know that he is part of your happiness.

Since most discussions of dieting and weight usually bring up feelings, remember that your husband's approach to emotions is likely to be different from yours. As a child, you probably had a girlfriend with whom you could share your deepest secrets. Now, as an adult, when you're upset, you call a friend and pour your heart out. Men don't usually do this. When he was a boy, your husband didn't get much experience talking about his feelings with his friends. Can you see him stopping a baseball game to discuss his hurt feelings after he struck out and another kid made fun of him?

Now, when you tell your husband how you are feeling, you hope that he will respond supportively. Instead he ignores you, changes the topic, or else goes into a lecture in which he tries to be helpful by providing all sorts of logical solutions to whatever you are discussing. Even if you have his attention, he completely misses how you are feeling. If you've been through this routine a few times, you may have given up talking with him about sensitive issues. With a little effort, you will be able to break through this impasse.

You Call 411, He Hears 911

Dr. Gottman's research suggests that men and women have different physiological responses when emotions are being discussed. You may be looking for reassurance, or calmly asking for information (like calling 411), yet his body responds as though it were an emergency. Your husband's blood pressure and heart rate will rise much higher than yours does. For you, it's just a conversation, while for him it sets off fire alarms and shrieking sirens inside his body. His attention is focused on silencing the alarms and sirens so that he can calm down. Most husbands try to accomplish this by tuning out what their wife is saying, getting up and leaving the room, or by yelling at her so she will leave. Unfortunately, neither his feelings, your feelings, nor the issue you were trying to discuss gets resolved.

If your husband hasn't had much experience talking about his own feelings, and his blood pressure goes up when you try to tell him about yours, how are the two of you possibly going to discuss how you feel about eating, gaining and losing weight, or any sensitive topic? Applying Dr. Gottman's strategies, here are five rules to help communication. Now, there are no guarantees that once you have mastered these strategies, the two of you will agree about everything (wouldn't that be boring?). Still, your discussions will be more satisfying and bring you closer, even when you don't see eye to eye.

Rule 1: Calm Yourself

Even if your husband experiences a more intense physical arousal than you do, you still may get worked up when you try to discuss your eating with him. Mentally you are anticipating being put down, ignored, or perhaps you expect him to talk down to you as though you were a child. You've been frustrated before, so you are preparing yourself, planning your arguments, bracing yourself for the bad feelings that are likely to result. Your body will respond to this type of thinking, and before long, your heart will be pounding and blood pumping. This is counter productive; you can't think clearly. If your husband should say something helpful, even if it comes in the middle of a lengthy tirade, you wouldn't be able to recognize that he is being helpful. Or if you're feeling attacked, you try to make yourself feel better by counterattacking. This results in an escalation of the conflict. Both of you are feeling bad and nothing has been accomplished.

Before you start any important discussion, make sure you are calm. If you start calm, but find yourself getting worked up, you can call a time-out and relax yourself before resuming the discussion. Box 9 presents a list of practical techniques that you can use to calm yourself.

Box 9. Calming Yourself

The trick to calming yourself is to change what is happening in your mind and your body. Start with your mind.

1. Instead of the usual negative thoughts ("How could he say that? Doesn't he realize . . ."), try to take a more detached, problem-solving view. For example, if your husband responds negatively to something you said, it may be that he really doesn't understand your point of view. Instead of being hurt, think how you can express yourself in a way that makes sense to him.

2. Don't get overwhelmed with negativity. Even if the discussion is getting heated, remind yourself of

some of your husband's positive qualities. Remember a specific example of the two of you having a good time together, or think of something he did that made you feel loving toward him.

3. Keep an argument in perspective. Remind yourself that you are two individuals with different backgrounds and experiences who are involved with each other. Some conflict is inevitable. Don't overgeneralize by interpreting a disagreement as evidence that you are incompatible.

Now, pay attention to your body.

1. Focus on your breathing. Take a long, deep breath. Completely fill your lungs with air until it feels as if they will burst. Hold the breath for a few seconds, then slowly exhale. Do it again. As you exhale, try to let some of your tension go.

2. Practice muscle relaxation. When you are stressed, your muscles become tight. You can learn to relax them. Call a time-out, lie down, or sit in a recliner that supports your whole body. Start with your hands and arms. Make a clenched fist and bend both arms so that all the muscles are tight. Feel the tension from your fingertips up to your shoulder, hold the tension for a few seconds, release your muscles, and relax. Let the relaxation develop for 30 seconds, and repeat. Then move on to your face and head. From your jaw and tongue to your nose, eyes, and scalp. Tighten all the muscles, hold the tension, release the tension, and relax. Repeat this tightening-holding-releasing-relaxing procedure throughout your body. Do your neck and shoulders, chest and stomach, buttocks, legs and feet. As you make your way down the body, make sure tension has not crept back into an area you've already

relaxed. With practice, you'll find that this process is easier, and takes less time to produce complete muscle relaxation.

Rule 2: Listen Without Becoming Defensive

Your husband isn't an enemy. Even when he is angry, try to interpret his anger as the product of the frustration he feels. He may be frustrated because he feels that an important message is not getting through to you. When he senses that you are making a genuine effort to understand him, even if you still don't agree with what he is saying, the anger will decrease. It isn't easy, but try to ignore the words or tone of voice that comes from his anger. Instead, imagine how you would feel if you were him right now. Let him know that you are paying attention and trying to see his point of view. Make sure that while he is talking, you don't look away, roll your eyes, or look at him like you think he's crazy. Make sure that your body language and facial expressions are telling him that you are listening respectfully to what he has to say. If he sees you listening and trying to understand, it will be more difficult for him to stay angry.

Rule 3: Complain, Don't Criticize

Any relationship is going to have some disagreements and disappointments. Would you really want to live with someone who agreed with everything you said? Although it sounds good, before long your relationship would be incredibly dull. It may not always be pleasant when two people express honest disagreement, but it is essential to make a relationship work. Two suggestions to make the inevitable disagreements more productive and less unpleasant are:

First, complain but don't criticize. You are complaining when you state your objections to a specific behavior or situation. When Jeff and Margaret were at a party and Jeff made fun of her diet, afterward Margaret said, "It really makes me angry when you make fun of my diets. Usually you say that you want me to lose weight, but when you ridicule me for trying, I don't know what to think."

A criticism is a more general, sweeping statement that usually communicates blame. For example, Margaret could have said, "You always make fun of me. No wonder that I get discouraged and give up." Whenever a statement of a problem includes the words "always" or "never," it's likely to be a criticism, not a complaint. When you complain, you are asking your husband to change a behavior. When you criticize, you are attacking him as a person so it's likely that he will try to defend himself. Complaining can produce desirable change; criticism will produce defensiveness, and probably a frustrating argument.

Second, try to keep a positive outlook even when you are discussing serious disagreements. Even when your husband is being incredibly irritating and refusing to understand your thoroughly reasonable point of view, try to remember some of his good qualities. If you can't think of any right now, what attracted you to him way back when? Do you like his sense of humor? Does he have a soft side, or some special quality that other people don't see which makes you feel close to him? Do you (or did you) admire the way he thinks? Even if you haven't seen some of these qualities for a while, try to place the current conflict in a larger perspective which includes them.

I'm not suggesting that you "put on a happy face" and forget about what's troubling you. On the contrary, you are wanting your husband to make some changes. When you recognize his positive qualities, and occasionally mention them to him, you are making it easier for him to change. If he feels admired and accepted, he can let his guard down, look nondefensively at his behavior, and begin to understand your viewpoint. Don't expect immediate results, but try to focus on the positive aspects of the relationship during your next serious discussion and see what happens.

Rule 4: Validate, Validate, Validate (and then Validate Some More)

Few things feel as good as being understood and accepted. Did you ever have a friend whom you could talk to about anything? You could be confused, or your thoughts were kind of crazy, it didn't matter. Your friend would listen respectfully and let you know that she or he could see how you felt. Your friend wasn't giving you advice, and might not have agreed with everything you were saying, but by letting you know that you were understood, you felt better. If you don't get that type of empathy from your husband, would you like it? Wouldn't it be nice if he really understood your struggles with weight? This will be one of our goals. It will be accomplished, in part, by providing him with information—from this book—that will help him understand. However, information by itself won't do the trick. He will need to know how you feel. You will teach him the emotional part of empathy. You can do this by demonstrating how it is done. Box 10 describes some simple methods for communicating empathy. You don't have to use the exact words that are printed on this page. When you understand the idea of communicating empathy you can use words that seem natural for you.

Box 10. Empathize

When you empathize with your husband, you put yourself in his shoes and imagine what it feels like to be him. Once you've got a picture of what it is like to be him—for example, how frustrated he must have felt, or how happy he must have been—then you let him know that you understand. Although it may seem artificial at first, there are several simple things you can do to communicate empathy. You can:

1. Repeat his feeling. Even if you don't agree, or think he should have done something different, acknowledge how he felt *(not* how you think he should have felt). You can do this with a simple statement like, "That must have been frustrating" or "I bet that was really stressful."

2. Show that you are with him. While he is expressing a feeling, look at him, nod occasionally, and say something like "uh-huh" or "mmm-hmm." This doesn't mean that you are necessarily agreeing with everything he says, but you are letting him know that you are interested, and emotionally, you are with him.

3. Ask for clarification. You have repeated his feeling and demonstrated that you are with him. Now, every so often, restate what you have heard and ask him if you understood correctly. This demonstrates that you are trying to understand, and if you are missing something, he has your permission to try to explain.

Rule 5: Practice Makes Perfect

If any or all of Rules 1–4 seem strange or unnatural, you may dismiss them as impractical or unrealistic. On the other hand, if they seem entirely reasonable or obvious, you may assume that, since you understand them, you must be using them. In both instances, you're likely to be wrong. All couples, even when one spouse is certifiably crazy, can profitably use these strategies. Even if you know this, when your husband is being his most infuriating self, it's difficult to remember to calm yourself first, then respond nondefensively with empathy.

Although the focus of this book is on weight loss, these five rules can help in communicating about other topics. Use them when you discuss household chores, finances, dealing with in-laws, or any other topic that is likely to produce disagreement. If there has been a lot of conflict in your marriage, practice these strategies when you are discussing a topic that isn't too controversial. You can expect to practice for quite some time until these responses become automatic. Still, if you're planning on spending a lifetime with your husband, you might as well start now.

Getting Started

Each chapter in Part II will have suggestions for involving your husband or there will be a short section for him to read. Your progress will not depend on his willingness to participate. Like Jeff, some husbands are hesitant at first and only get involved after you have made progress on your own. Other husbands participate enthusiastically in some steps, but don't get involved in others. Since I don't know how your husband will respond to each of the steps, I will also suggest how you can proceed with each if your husband is not interested.

To start, ask your husband to read the letter on page 91, when it is convenient. If he resists, or if he agrees but doesn't follow through, wait two or three days and ask again. If, at the end of a week, he still hasn't read the letter, you can assume that he is not going to participate. Keeping calm (Rule 1), complain about his lack of support without criticizing him (Rule 3). Let him know that you are going to proceed without him, but since he has chosen not to participate, you will expect him to avoid commenting on your weight, or what you are eating. If he makes a comment anyway, either suggest again that he read the relevant part of the book, or feel free to ignore the comment until he does so.

A Note for Your Husband

Dear Husband,

Your wife is showing you this book because she wants you to understand the weight control program she is starting. You may be a little skeptical, or even completely mistrusting. Although I don't know the details of your specific situation, I do know that many husbands are tired of listening to their wife's constant preoccupation with diets, low-calorie foods, weight loss programs, exercise tapes and equipment which are sometimes expensive but never seem to accomplish much. After several years of diets which go nowhere, many husbands "tune out" when their wife starts talking about weight.

Some husbands are sympathetic to their wife's concern with weight but question why she has so much trouble dieting. For many men, controlling their weight is straightforward. They can usually keep a stable weight, and if they do find that they've gained, they can cut back on their eating until they lose the new weight. If this has been your experience, it's difficult to understand why your wife is constantly struggling with her weight.

Regardless of your experience, this book will help you understand your wife's difficulty with weight. Why is this important? Research shows that husbands can have a significant impact on the success of their wife's weight loss. Several years ago a review of 12 studies comparing programs with husband participation to similar programs that did not involve the husband found that the programs with husbands' involvement had significantly better results.[35] These findings do not mean that you have to go on a diet, or that you are responsible for what your wife eats, but rather that your wife will benefit from your help, support, and encouragement.

A husband is in a unique position to offer support. Groups like Weight Watchers or Overeaters Anonymous can provide support, but this is not as effective. You eat many of your meals with her and will be with her as she makes many of the changes necessary for permanent weight control. Your encouragement, at the time she is following the program, will be far more powerful than any support she may get, later on, from a weight loss group. By participating, you will help ensure that the changes she makes are permanent so that she can maintain her weight loss indefinitely.

There are many reasons for helping your wife lose weight. In addition to having a healthier, more attractive wife, your marriage may get stronger and the two of you may have a better time together. When a women loses weight, usually it leads to increased self-esteem, which can improve the quality of a marriage. One study found that after weight loss, women became more involved in social activities with their husbands, increased their participation in physical activities with him, and had more satisfying sexual relations.[36] Your involvement should benefit both of you.

While it is not necessary for you to read the whole

book, you are certainly welcome to do so. If you don't want to read it all, there are several sections that may answer specific questions that you have. If you're confused about all the hype about the fat gene, or low-fat diets, look at Chapter 2, which deals with some of the causes of obesity. Chapter 1 describes differences between men and women when it comes to weight, while Chapter 3 explains how the changes that come with being married and raising a family contribute to weight gain. Part II presents the changes she will make so that she can gradually, but permanently, lose weight. Your wife will read these chapters and determine when she would like your help. She will either ask you to read the relevant sections or describe the methods and ask you for help making specific changes. If you don't think that you can participate, there will be directions for her to do that assignment without you. Keep in mind that you are not responsible for the success or failure of the program, but you can help.

If you have been concerned about your own weight, or even if you've just noticed that your stomach isn't as flat as it used to be, this could be a good time for you to change your eating and exercise habits. Research suggests that overweight husbands participating in their wife's weight control program can lose a significant amount of weight.[37] It will be easier for both of you to make the changes necessary to lose weight if you are working together and supporting each other. Still, if you are not motivated to lose, you should not feel that you are required to participate. A diet that is only a response to pressure from others won't work.

Whether or not you decide to lose weight, you can still support your wife's efforts by:

1. Showing interest in what she is doing. When

your wife asks you to read a few pages, try to do it as soon as possible.

2.   Being positive. No dieter is perfect. Instead of criticizing or pointing out her mistakes, notice when she has followed the program and compliment her for it.

3.   Don't focus on weight. Weight loss doesn't always proceed smoothly. If your wife is following the program, she deserves your support regardless of what the scale says.

4.   Don't tempt her. Try not to eat fattening foods in front of your wife, and if you do, definitely don't offer her any.

I hope you'll try to help your wife when she asks for your participation. I think you will be pleased with the results.

PART II

A Recipe for Losing Weight and Improving Your Relationship

CHAPTER 5

No More Yo-Yos

This isn't your first attempt to lose weight. How many different diets, programs, and methods have you tried? By now you're a little skeptical about any program that claims you can lose weight and keep it off. Maybe you've read that all diets are doomed to failure—even if you lose weight, it is inevitable that you will regain it. Yet each time you see the cover of a magazine with a headline describing a diet that promises easy weight loss, there's a little curiosity—could this be the diet that finally works for me? The first ingredient in the Recipe for Losing Weight and Improving Your Relationship is understanding and making peace with your dieting history.

What's Wrong with this Picture?

Humorist Art Buchwald said that the word "diet" comes from the verb "to die." Amy, a 30-year-old, 175-pound mother of two, would definitely agree. In our first session, Amy reviewed her dieting history. I will spare you the details of all the diets she's tried and all the slow, painful "deaths" she has suffered. Instead I'll just describe her typical pattern.

Since she was 18, Amy made at least one major dieting attempt each year. Sometimes it was a commercial program like Weight Watchers or Nutri/systems; other times she bought a diet best-seller and tried to follow the menus. Her enthusiasm and serious involvement lasted anywhere between 3 days (a vegetarian diet that she absolutely hated) to 18 weeks on a program conducted at a local medical clinic. On most diets she lost some weight, usually less than 10 pounds, but occasionally as much as 30 pounds. Regardless of her success, or how long she was able to maintain her enthusiasm, eventually it waned. Sometimes a craving was her downfall. Especially when she was feeling lonely, the desire for her favorite treats was impossible to ignore. She resisted as long as she could, but eventually she gave in and then became discouraged and gave up. Other times there was no particular emotional upset but just a small change in routine. For example, one of the times she belonged to Weight Watchers, she did well as long as she maintained perfect attendance. When she missed a meeting because of back-to-school night, she found it harder to go to the next meeting. Although she pushed herself to go, it didn't have the urgency it once did. Still, she would go to the meetings even though she was slacking off on the program between meetings. Eventually she felt embarrassed because she wasn't losing any more weight. So she stopped attending, felt like a failure, and started to regain the weight she had lost.

When Amy dieted on her own, the diet lasted for a shorter period. Since the diet book cost less than the commercial programs, she didn't feel the same level of commitment. Also, without the meetings, fewer people knew that she was trying to lose weight. It was easier to give up since she would not feel as much social pressure and embarrassment explaining that she had failed again.

After the failure of a diet or program, Amy would get very discouraged. She felt she was doomed to fail at any attempt to lose weight. Since she "went off" her diet, there was nothing preventing Amy from eating all the forbidden foods that she had missed while on the diet. Sometimes she would feel out of control as she ate huge amounts of ice cream, pizza, Oreos, and all the goodies that she had missed. She looked down, with a guilty expression on her face, as she told me about her post-diet binges. I had the feeling that she expected that I was going to lecture her, giving her a well-deserved scolding for being such a bad girl.

After a period of guilty bingeing, Amy would settle into a pattern of eating in which she ate most of the foods she wanted with an occasional attempt to avoid a few "bad" foods. Throughout this stage she had a continuous sense that she should be more careful about what she ate. Frequently she felt guilty because she was eating foods that were fattening, but she usually went ahead and ate them anyway. This stage continued for several months until her bad feelings and weight gain escalated to the point where she felt that she had to do something. As the pressure mounted, she would pay more attention to diets or programs that were featured on TV or in a magazine until she felt the urge to start another diet. Then the sequence would start again.

Does any of this sound familiar? Have you gone through the repeated yo-yo diet cycle (sometimes called the rhythm method of girth control)? To better understand the problems with dieting, let's look closely at Amy's yo-yo pattern. Her weight loss attempts followed a six-step sequence:

1. Initial enthusiasm and commitment
2. Adherence to the diet or program

3. Slipping after an emotional upset or a change in routine

4. Recognition that the program had failed

5. An "oh what the hell" period when Amy ate anything she wanted and gained

6. Reaching or exceeding her original weight, she became frightened and started "watching" her weight.

What Is a Diet?

Before we go any further, before starting any new weight loss program, it is necessary to understand the reasons for your lack of success with earlier efforts. Forgive me if I sound like a psychology professor, but let's start with the definition of dieting. You cut down on your food, especially high-fat, high-calorie foods so that you'll lose weight. Right? Unfortunately, there is more to dieting than eating less. According to psychologists Kelly Brownell and Judith Rodin, in addition to restricting your eating, dieting usually includes feelings of deprivation and a set of thoughts about your weight, food, and exercise.[38] In other words, when you go on a diet, your thinking and feelings are also changed, usually for the worse.

While you can see the changes in your eating (no more pepperoni pizza), the changes in your thoughts and feelings are much less obvious. When you diet, you feel bad and have unhelpful thoughts. Learning to check your thoughts and feelings, and keep a positive mind-set while on a diet, is very important. Ultimately, changing your thoughts and feelings will be as important as controlling the food you eat. I've listed on the next page some of the most common types of negative thoughts associated with dieting. As you read through the list, recall a recent diet and see if you had similar thoughts. Put a check mark in the space after a diet thought that you've had:

1.   Dieting is like a light switch—it is either on or off. When I am on a diet, I am always restricting my eating; when I am off my diet, I don't need to watch what I eat._____

2.   Dieting is always painful. When I am on a diet, I am continuously aware that I have been deprived of my favorite foods, and I frequently feel hunger pangs._____

3.   Diets never work, especially for me. Despite the hype, even when I am enthusiastically getting started, a little voice inside says, "Who are you fooling? You know you can't lose weight."_____

4.   I have to be hard on myself to diet. Hating the way I look and being angry with myself whenever I slip is necessary to keep me motivated to stay on my diet._____

5.   It's unfair that I have to diet. Other people can eat whatever they want. Why should I be deprived of my favorite foods?_____

6.   I've always failed at diets. Even when I lose weight, I'm still not able to reach my goal._____

7.   Since I have trouble dieting, I have (choose one, or more): no willpower, no self-discipline, a weak character, a personality defect, a neurosis, unconscious conflicts about dependency needs, a lack of moral fiber, etc., etc., etc._____

Are any of these thoughts familiar? Go back and look at the thoughts you have checked. How do you feel after you think about yourself and your diet in these terms? Any, or all of these thoughts will produce bad feelings. For example, if you think you have no willpower, you will feel guilty. If you think that you need to be hard on yourself, your self-esteem will suffer. If you think you always fail, you will feel guilty and depressed, while if you think you are being deprived, you will feel angry or frustrated. Now, how long can you go on doing something that undermines your self-esteem and makes you feel guilty, depressed, angry, and frustrated? It's only a matter of time before you'll give up doing anything that makes you feel that bad. To summarize, in addition to controlling eating, being on a diet includes typical "diet thoughts" which produce unpleasant emotions. Even if controlling your eating was easy, these emotions would eventually become unbearable so you still would give up the diet to feel better.

Changing Your Thinking About Dieting

Losing weight does not require that you think painful thoughts and feel bad. The first ingredient in your Recipe for Losing Weight is to change your thoughts and feelings so that you can comfortably lose weight. You can do this by first understanding why most diet thoughts are irrational, and then substituting more sensible alternatives. You may have to practice by reminding yourself of the rational thoughts several times a day, but you will find the bad feelings decreasing as the new thoughts take hold. Pay particular attention to the thoughts you checked. Look at each of the diet thoughts critically and consider the more rational alternative:

1. Dieting is not an on or off switch. People who successfully lose weight, and a large number of people who are not overweight but want to prevent the weight gain that comes with aging (see Reason 2 in Chapter 2), control what they eat. Sometimes they are more active and they deliberately work at avoiding certain

foods (at a party, for example), while other times they have developed habits (shopping, serving food) that enable them to control their food consumption without a conscious effort. They aren't on or off a diet; they have developed an ongoing lifestyle that promotes weight control.

2.   Watching what you eat doesn't have to be a continuous struggle. For example, learning to deal with emotional states that produce cravings (see Chapter 1) will make the cravings less intense. Also, there is some evidence that people who lose weight and keep it off for a year or more may find that they have less of an appetite and fewer cravings for sweets.[39] With planning, you will be able to substitute foods, alter routines, and decrease your reliance on food to nurture yourself so that it doesn't feel like you are always hungry or struggling with temptation.

3.   It is true that those ads you see in tabloids, women's magazines, and drugstore products promising "quick, effortless" weight loss are totally unrealistic. You may have also seen an often repeated estimate that 95 percent of all dieters will regain any weight they might be lucky enough to lose. Even though this figure comes from a reputable scientific study,[40] the data for this study were collected in the 1950s. Since then behavioral methods have been developed, and our knowledge of nutrition and exercise has increased greatly. A *Consumer Reports* survey of 19,000 people in commercial programs like Weight Watchers and Jenny Craig found that at least 25 percent were able to lose weight and keep it off for more than two years.[41] Most people usually diet on their own before trying a commercial program. One study suggests that 62 percent are able to lose weight without joining a diet program.[42] Whatever the actual number of successful dieters is, it is clear that losing weight, and keeping it off, is possible. Changing your

thinking and getting support from your husband will greatly increase your likelihood of success.

4.   Hating yourself, or even hating the way that you look, does not increase your motivation to lose weight. Research shows that overeating is more common among dieters with low self-esteem than among those who like themselves.[43] Imagine that after dinner, you go back in the kitchen, open the refrigerator, find the leftover pie, and eat a piece. You feel guilty, you think, "What a pig I am," or "I'm a slob with no willpower," or some equally negative statement about yourself. This type of put-down chips away at your self-esteem and does *nothing* to help you to deal with your cravings the next time you are tempted. Instead of punishing yourself, acknowledge that you made a mistake and try to figure out what you can do to prevent it from happening again. Develop a plan so that you don't have the pie next time (see Box 11 for a few ideas) and then allow yourself to feel good when you have avoided it. Focus on being nice to yourself when you accomplish your goals rather than punishing yourself when you fall short.

5.   It might be unfair that you are not one of the few lucky people who never need to watch what they eat. It is also unfair that some people are born blind or deaf. If you are going to compare yourself to others, recognize that a genetic tendency to gain weight easily is not the worst possible handicap.

Box 11. Living Dangerously

If you have snack foods or high-calorie desserts in your home, you are living dangerously since they present continuous temptation. If you really need chocolate, go to the nearest convenience store and buy a

single serving, but don't keep it in the house. If you
need dessert for guests:

1. Buy the dessert on the day you are having the
guests and buy only as much as you will need.
2. If you should have any leftovers, send them home
with your guests.
3. If your guests refuse to take the leftovers, throw
them out.
4. If you can't make yourself throw food in the garbage, immediately put it in the back of the freezer.
Hopefully you will forget about it until it is covered with
ice and then you can throw it away when you clean out
the freezer.

6. Most dieters set unrealistic goals for themselves.
Sometimes they expect to lose weight too quickly ("I
need to lose 10 pounds before my vacation next week"),
sometimes their goal weight is impossible ("I want to
fit into a size 5"), and sometimes the goals are both
too quick and impossible ("I want to fit into a size 5 by
Friday"). If you have never reached your goal, it may
be that the way you set your goal was impractical. In the
next chapter, you will learn how to use the information
presented in Chapters 2 and 3 to set goals that make
sense for you.

7. Anytime you make a broad, sweeping generaliza-
tion about your personality, you are likely to be wrong.
The only people who diet effortlessly, who never have
any difficulties or setbacks, are the people lucky enough
to never need to diet. If you are going to control your
weight, there will be times when nothing seems to be
working. Even if this is a frequent occurrence,
explaining these difficulties in terms of a permanent

moral or psychological defect doesn't help. Giving your-self a label implies that there is nothing you can do about it—you are doomed because of your personality or character. Instead, you will learn how to become a detective and solve the mystery of your dieting downfalls. Once you know the cause, you will be able to do some-thing different. This is more productive than deciding that you have no willpower and giving up.

When Amy and I discussed her thoughts about dieting, she recognized that some of her thinking was irrational, but she still found it hard to not feel bad about her diets. She was fighting with herself. On one hand, she knew that she was being unrealistic, but she couldn't make peace with herself. She continued to feel bad about dieting. Why were her negative feelings so deeply ingrained? Like most overweight people in our culture, deep inside, Amy knew that she was a sinner.

The Morality of Dieting

Gluttony is a sin. Being slender is an outward sign of virtue, but if you are fat, your body is tangible proof that you are a sinner. Most sinning occurs in private, but not eating. Even if you ate all your meals by yourself, everyone would know that you are a sinner because you're not thin. If this sounds far-fetched, why do advertisers of fattening desserts refer to them as "sinful"? Why did Weight Watch-ers categorize some foods as "illegal"? Why are you "good" if you follow your diet, but "bad" if you don't? Whether you are religious or not, traditional notions of sin influence the way you think about your weight and diet.

Confusing eating with morality has a long history in America. For example, in the 1830s health reformer

Sylvester Graham (the popularizer of graham crackers) referred to gluttony as "the greatest of all causes of evil." John Harvey Kellogg, the founder of the cereal company bearing his name, claimed that "mental and moral inefficiency" could be traced to the kitchen.[44] Although these ideas may strike you as old-fashioned, they still exert a powerful influence. Why else would you feel so bad when you don't follow your diet?

When I discussed this with Amy, she adamantly denied that she was immoral because her diets were unsuccessful; instead she attributed her bad feelings to health concerns:

> *I don't think I'm a sinner who's going to hell because I blew my diet. That's ridiculous. The reason I feel bad is because I know that it's unhealthy for me to weigh 175 pounds, and I know I should be able to do something about it.*

Although this seems to be a perfectly logical argument (you agree with Amy, don't you?), being "unhealthy" doesn't account for Amy's (or your) bad feelings. If it was only your health concerns that caused the negative emotions, you would feel equally guilty when you drive without wearing your seat belt. When was the last time you called yourself a slob or questioned your willpower because you forgot to buckle your seat belt? You also know that if you sit in the sun too long, you increase the risk of skin cancer. When you get a sunburn, do you berate yourself for having no self-discipline, or being weak or lazy? Every day there are health risks that you could avoid, but you don't bother. If your husband reminds you to buckle your seat belt or use sunscreen when you go to the beach, you can agree or disagree, but there isn't any implication that you are immoral. Only eating makes you feel so bad.

In order to succeed at weight loss, you will have to change your thoughts and feelings about dieting. *You will have to view dieting with the same rational, emotionally neutral*

perspective as you view wearing a seat belt or using sunscreen.
When you can think about your food choices without guilt,
shame, and moral judgments, you will be able to lose
weight. Now, go back to pages 102–106, and review the
seven rational thoughts about dieting. Think about each
one and see if you can make it fit for you. Repeat them
out loud. Find the ideas that are hardest to accept, write
them down on a Post-it note, and put it in your appointment book, on your dresser, your mirror, or anyplace that
you look at frequently. Do whatever you have to do to
challenge your old, irrational way of thinking about diets
and weight. Accept the fact that, regardless of your weight
or diet history, you are not a sinner. Box 12 presents a few
suggestions to help.

Box 12. Be Good to Yourself

Many women allow the ups and downs of their weight
to determine their mood for the day and their self-
esteem. In addition to creating bad feelings and a poor
self-concept, overemphasizing the significance of your
weight is counterproductive when you are trying to lose
weight. Having healthy self-esteem and mostly positive
moods will increase your motivation. To improve self-
esteem:

1. Make a list of your positive attributes, skills, and
talents. Since you are not going to show this to anyone,
don't worry about being conceited or immodest. Are
you trustworthy and honest? Do you have a good sense
of humor? Are you a good friend, a hard worker, intelli-
gent, creative, artistic, or musical? Can you teach, draw
blood, type, paint, garden, write computer programs,
tune automobiles, or sew well? Remember that you
tend to take for granted many of your skills since you

have been doing them without problems for some time. Even if you don't think that your skills are a big deal, imagine how long it would take someone else to learn to do them as well as you do, and then give yourself credit for having already done them. Keep your list with you and take it out several times a day to remind yourself of some of your good qualities.

2. After each success, regardless of whether you've turned in a lengthy report at work, or just cleaned the kitchen and polished the silverware, stop and give yourself a verbal pat on the back. You are not being narcissistic, and as long as you don't make unflattering comparisons to other people, you are not being conceited. You did something worthwhile; you deserve to enjoy your success and take pride in your accomplishment.

3. When someone compliments you, agree with him! When your boss says, "You did a good job," instead of responding with, "It was no big deal," you can say something like, "Thanks, I think it went well." You are not bragging, but you are letting yourself and others know that you did well.

Is Your Husband Living in Sin?

Like everyone else, husbands tend to see weight and dieting as moral issues. Since he is involved, it will be helpful if he learns to think about weight loss as habit change, without the implications of moral judgment. Here are several ways you can help him to do this:

1. Make sure that you understand and accept that what you eat is not a moral issue or a direct reflection

of your worth as a person. When you are clear on the concept, pay attention to your language and emotions when you discuss weight with your husband. Do you use value-laden terms such as "being good" or "cheat" or "lazy" to describe your eating and exercise behaviors? When you use these words, you are implicitly accepting the moral view of weight. What about your body language? Do you hang your head, avoid eye contact, or look ashamed when you talk about diet and weight? Instead, when you discuss your eating, use neutral terms and accept responsibility for your behavior without guilt. For example, you could say, "I decided to have that leftover piece of pie," rather than "I cheated."

2.   When the topic comes up, tell your husband that eating is not a sin and feeling bad will not help you lose weight. If he is interested, show him the relevant parts of this chapter. Explain that losing weight will take considerable effort over a long time period and it is unlikely that you will do it perfectly. Ask him to offer sincere praise when he sees you making good choices, but to avoid the temptation to nag if you are not. In the long run, feeling good about yourself will help you maintain the persistence necessary for success.

3.   Are there any activities that your husband would like you to do with him, but you don't because you think you are too fat? Don't worry about how you would look. Don't be self-conscious if you are not as agile as you would like to be; go ahead and do them anyway. Let your husband know that your change of heart is part of the Recipe for Losing Weight.

Dieting Is Hard Work; Be Good to Yourself

Do you know how to drive a car with a manual transmission? Try to remember how you learned. For every smooth start there were several times you stalled, bucked, or peeled rubber. Can you type without looking at the keyboard? Remember the pages filled with errors when you were learning. Anytime you learn a new skill or change a long-standing habit, progress is uneven. There are days when nothing seems to go right, and you wonder if you'll ever improve. Sometimes it seems more reasonable just to give up.

Learning the behaviors necessary for permanent weight loss takes more effort than driving a stick shift or typing since you will be changing some well-entrenched behaviors that occur all day long, not just when you're in the car or at your desk. Even though you are making an effort, there will be times when you forget and the old behavior will return. Other times, you'll be aware of what you are doing, but you just don't have the energy to substitute the new behavior for the old. Don't despair—you can inoculate yourself against these setbacks.

Psychologist Roy Baumeister has done extensive studies of how people control their own behavior. He concluded that self-regulation is a limited resource; there's only so much you can do at any time. When you are tired or stressed, making yourself feel better "uses up" the energy that could have gone to control other behaviors.[45] To make your habit change easier, allow yourself to have fun when you are not focused on your eating. Enjoying yourself and feeling good will recharge your batteries so you will have more energy to devote to the Recipe. You won't feel as deprived when you forgo a tempting food if you have recently experienced rewards other than food.

Unfortunately I usually encounter resistance when I suggest to a patient who is working on her weight that she make a deliberate effort to have fun. The idea that you don't deserve to enjoy yourself because you haven't achieved your goal is a direct consequence of the fat = sin thinking. Remember, you are not a sinner, so you don't need to be miserable to redeem yourself.

Think about fun activities that you have put off until you lose weight. Listed below are a few activities that patients have told me they won't do until they reach their goal:

- Buy new clothes
- Go to a class reunion
- Dance
- Ride a bicycle
- Have sex with the lights on
- Go on a trip
- Get undressed in front of their husbands

Buying clothes is probably the most commonly post-poned pleasure. Many overweight women won't buy themselves new clothes until they reach their goal. Since it may take months to get to their goal, they deprive themselves of shopping, which is an activity they would enjoy, and feel even worse about their looks. So, in addition to the usual unhappiness about being overweight, you are dissatisfied with an old, unflattering wardrobe. This does not help motivate you to make the effort that is necessary for habit change. Instead, to the extent your budget allows, enjoy the pleasure of shopping for new clothes. You don't need to be extravagant and buy a whole new wardrobe, but you might feel better if there were a few outfits that you enjoyed wearing. If you are concerned that any clothes that you buy now will be too big when you have lost weight, you can still buy fashionable shoes, purses, or accessories now. You don't need to feel deprived while you are losing weight.

What have you put off until you've lost weight? Is there anything your husband would like you to do with him, but you feel you can't until you're thinner? In the following spaces, list activities that you would like to do but have postponed because of your weight:

1. _____ 3. _____

2. _____ 4. _____

What are you waiting for? Go ahead and start with the activity that would be the easiest to do.

Stopping the Yo-Yo

Remember Amy, the 30-year-old yo-yo dieter? After some discussion, she was able to change her diet thinking, get beyond the fat = sin thinking, and allow herself a few pleasures that she had been postponing. The up and down, up and down yo-yo stopped. She wasn't perfect. There were periods where her adherence decreased, but this was different from the "oh what the hell" periods when she was a yo-yo dieter. Figure 2 compares Amy's yo-yoing with the lifestyle change resulting from the Recipe for Losing Weight. Once you have been able to give up yo-yo dieting, you shouldn't expect perfect adherence to the Recipe for Losing Weight, or any other weight loss program. Like Amy, you should expect some times when your adherence weakens. For example, during a particularly stressful period at work, or during the weeks between Thanksgiving and New Year's, you might find yourself slipping, but this will be a temporary interruption that you will learn to handle in Chapter 13. When things ease up at work, or after January 1, you can pick up where you left off without the bad feelings and self-defeating behaviors of the yo-yo cycle.

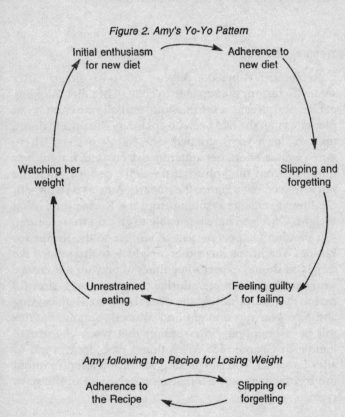

Figure 2. Amy's Yo-Yo Pattern

Initial enthusiasm for new diet → Adherence to new diet → Slipping and forgetting → Feeling guilty for failing → Unrestrained eating → Watching her weight → Initial enthusiasm for new diet

Amy following the Recipe for Losing Weight

Adherence to the Recipe ⇄ Slipping or forgetting

CHAPTER 6

Ready, Set, Goal

The second ingredient in the Recipe has three parts: determining your readiness for permanent weight control, increasing self-awareness, and finding your personalized weight goal. Even if these seem obvious to you ("Of course I'm ready, I wouldn't be reading this book if I wasn't; I know I eat too much, and my goal is clear, I want to lose weight"), don't skip to the next chapter; humor me for a few pages.

Are You Ready?

There is no point in starting another program if the odds are stacked against you. While later chapters will include techniques for overcoming obstacles to weight loss, it is helpful now to honestly appraise your situation. Listed on page 116 are several prerequisites to successful weight loss. Although it may help to discuss these prerequisites with your husband, you are the only one who can decide if you are ready. Read each requirement and determine your readiness for change.

1. Your life is relatively stable now. The stresses and pressures of normal life sometimes make weight control more difficult, but not impossible. On the other hand, if an earthquake has just demolished your house, or if you have lost your job, had a death in the family, or moved to the other side of the country, your attention might be completely focused on the resulting turmoil. Remember Dr. Baumeister's admonition that self-regulation takes energy. You probably won't have the energy necessary for weight loss if you are spending all your time getting your life back together after a major upset.

2. Binge eating is not a routine for you. A binge is usually defined as the consumption of a very large amount of food in a short period of time. This is different from excess snacking or eating large portions because the binge eater usually feels that her eating is totally out of control. For example, overeating at Thanksgiving usually isn't a binge because it is a leisurely meal and you have some control over your eating. Research suggests that binge eaters have more difficulty losing weight and may be depressed. Although we will deal with some of the emotional causes of binge eating in Chapters 7 and 9, if you are a frequent binger, counseling may be helpful.

3. Increased activity is a possibility for you. Very few overweight women like the idea of exercise. After reading Chapter 12, you'll understand where your bad feelings come from, and what to do to become more comfortable with physical activity. At this point, even if you are not happy about it, you can accept the need to increase your activity level.

4. You are willing to try new behaviors. Although

the fantasy of "quick, effortless" weight loss sounds good, the reality is that, even if it were possible, you would quickly and effortlessly regain the weight unless you had also changed your eating and exercise habits. I am always perplexed when a patient tells me how unhappy she is, and then proceeds to tell me why she will continue to do whatever it was that made her so unhappy. To lose weight, you will not need superhuman willpower, but you will need to do something different from what you are doing now. It will not be exceptionally difficult or painful, but it might strike you as inconvenient.

Do you meet these four prerequisites? If you do, you are ready to proceed. If not, estimate a date in the future when you will have resolved the situations that are holding you back. Mark your calendar with this date so that you can reevaluate your readiness for change.

Getting to Know You

Knowing yourself is difficult when it comes to the seemingly obvious behavior of eating. Even experienced dieters who can recite the caloric value and fat content of most foods have difficulty accurately recalling their eating at the end of the day. For example, standing over the stove tasting the spaghetti sauce to see if it needs salt does not always register as eating. Research suggests that anything you do to increase your awareness of eating will result in less eating. Box 13 presents a simple method for monitoring your eating.

Box 13. Increasing Self-Awareness

The simplest, most efficient way of increasing awareness of your eating is to write down what you eat. To do this, get a 3 x 5 card and make four columns to record:

- The time the food was eaten.
- The type of food.
- The quantity of food (you don't need to measure the portion size precisely, just approximate).
- The grams of fat (if you don't know the fat content of the foods you eat, you can get this information from food labels or you can buy a small fat gram booklet at most supermarkets).

Try to do your recording either before or right after eating. If you wait until the end of the day, it's likely that you'll forget something. In social situations you can wait until the meal is over and you have some privacy before recording your consumption. Self-monitoring should not be embarrassing. It is important that you don't feel that your eating records will be evaluated by anyone, no matter how sincere their desire to help.

If your husband is participating, show him the "Note for Your Husband" in this chapter. Let him know that you will be keeping track of your eating and show him the form you will use. Make sure he understands that, unless you've asked him to, he is not supposed to review or supervise your self-monitoring. If you think it would help, you can ask him to remind you with a simple, single question like, "Are you going to monitor your eating today?" This can be done a *Maximum* of once per day. Any more is nagging, which is not helpful. On the other hand, he can be helpful by giving you "strokes" when he sees you writing on the 3 x 5 cards. The self-monitoring habit can take some time to establish. His support and encouragement can help.

Stop for a second and examine your thoughts as you were reading about self-monitoring. Are you skeptical about this assignment? Let's look at some of your objections. Yes, it is a bit of a chore to remember to carry a 3 x 5 card with you, but you remember to take your keys with you every day. If you fold the card in half and put it in your purse, wallet, or pocket it shouldn't be difficult to remember. Perhaps you feel that writing will interrupt the "natural flow" of eating. It will, but this is good! Stopping to write gives you a chance to make a conscious, deliberate decision about eating. You can ask yourself, "Do I really want this food, or am I just eating it because it's there?" If you really want it, go ahead, write it down, then eat it. If you decide you don't want it, you have given yourself the opportunity not to eat it.

In my experience with self-monitoring, the biggest problem is not forgetting or the unnaturalness of recording what you eat; it is that you will have a permanent record if you eat something "bad." If you are ashamed or feel guilty, you'd prefer to forget about it as soon as possible. You certainly won't want written evidence of your transgression. This discomfort is a direct consequence of thinking about eating as a sin. If you still feel this way, you will need to do more work to change your thoughts about weight and dieting. Go back and review "The Morality of Dieting" in Chapter 5. Even if you write "hot fudge sundae with whipped cream and cherries" on your 3 x 5 card, you are not a sinner.

Why am I making such a big deal about self-monitoring? Psychologists Raymond Baker and Daniel Kirschenbaum have demonstrated that dieters who monitor their eating lose more than dieters who don't. When dieters were given instructions to record their eating, they lost much more weight during weeks when they monitored than during weeks when they slacked off. Drs. Baker and Kirschenbaum think that dieters quit monitoring because they have unreasonably high standards.[46] When they aren't "perfect," it is too painful to think about the food they ate (or the "sin" they committed) so they give up monitoring, at least for the rest of the day. While I am not expecting perfection in monitoring (or anything else, for that matter), you will be more successful if you are consistent in self-monitoring.

Setting Your Goals

Have you ever been told, "You have such a pretty face; if you only lost weight, you'd be a real knockout?" Most yo-yo dieters have had fantasies about how wonderful life would be if only they were slim. For example, Melissa, a 19-year-old college junior, told me about her plans for the future. After graduating, she would go to business school to earn an M.B.A. degree. She would meet a handsome, ambitious fellow student, and they would fall in love and get married. Melissa's fantasy specified that her future husband would be "on the fast track" so that within a matter of years he would become an executive in a large firm. He would then be able to buy a nice home in an exclusive suburb, his and hers Mercedes-Benz's (she wanted a convertible), and take summer vacations in Europe and winter trips to the Caribbean. Meanwhile she would have given up her career so that she could stay home to raise their two perfect children. All of this would be possible only when she lost 30 pounds. For Melissa, her whole future was riding on achieving her weight loss goal. With so much riding on the outcome, each diet, and frequently each meal, became a stressful ordeal.

Melissa's 30-pound goal was based on comments an ex-boyfriend made when she was thinner ("You'd be real cute if you lost a little weight"), a number she found in a height-weight chart she saw in a magazine, and a whole set of unrealistic expectations. Even though she was constantly preoccupied with dieting, she never did reach her weight goal and usually felt like a failure. With a more realistic goal, she could have lost weight, even if her fantasy of the perfect life was not fulfilled.

Being Reasonable

When you have dieted before, how did you decide what your goal would be? Was it based on admonitions from your doctor, comments from your mother, or not-to-subtle "jokes" from your husband, all intended to let you know what they think you should weigh? Recognize that, despite pressure (subtle or not so subtle) from others, you are the only one who can set meaningful weight goals.

If you weren't influenced by others, did you use a height and weight chart, or use the weight that you thought would be necessary for a specific purpose (e.g., fit into an outfit, look as thin as an old friend)? These are all external criteria that don't take into account your uniqueness as an individual, including your age and possible inherited characteristics. You will find it easier to lose weight if you have a goal that makes sense for you. Let's start by considering your reasons for losing weight. Even if they don't include an M.B.A. and a Mercedes-Benz, you probably want to improve your appearance and health.

Thin = Beautiful

When you let yourself daydream, how do you see yourself? Are you on a beach wearing a sexy bikini, or at a party in a size 5 dress? Heads turn and you win admiring glances as you walk by. Okay, you can stop daydreaming. Although you know that these fantasies are unrealistic, they may have influenced how you have set your weight loss goals in the past. Even if your thinking about your weight has not been as unrealistic as Melissa's, there is no way to escape the influence of contemporary American culture. Current standards of beauty, based on models and actresses as ideals, require that a woman's body fat be limited to between 10 to 15 percent of her weight. Not only is this unrealistic, it is below the average range (between 22 to 25 percent) for healthy women of normal weight.[47]

The idea that thin is beautiful is a recent development. A hundred years ago, dimpled flesh ("cellulite") was beautiful while being skinny was associated with illness. Have you seen pinups of Marilyn Monroe? Calendars with her scantily clad body graced the walls of barber shops and garages throughout the 1950s and 1960s. Compare her physique with those of more recent sex symbols like Cindy Crawford or Julia Roberts. If you look closely at the Marilyn Monroe pinups, you'll see a hint of a double chin and thighs that would be unacceptable by current standards. Some feminists have suggested that while different shapes have been desirable during different historical periods, the one constant is that the ideal is unnatural and difficult to attain.[48] Regardless of the current standard, I have a more basic question: Are you sure that you'd want to be beautiful?

Stop for a moment and imagine what your life would be like if magically you could become thin and beautiful. Do you think your life would significantly improve? Here are several points to consider:

1.   If you had to be beautiful in order to find love or a sexual partner, the human race would have died out many years ago. Most people are average looking yet manage to find partners, have kids, and experience real love.

2.   People who are physically beautiful are not necessarily sexy. Even people who are perceived as beautiful

and sexy may suffer from sexual dysfunctions. Twenty years ago I worked in a medical school sex clinic. I recall one very attractive couple (she was a Playboy bunny) who had difficulty with their sexual relationship despite their love for each other. As we will see in Chapter 8, the brain is the most important sex organ regardless of your facial features or the shape of your body. Being beautiful does not guarantee that you will be sexually responsive or even enjoy sex.

3.   When they were children and adolescents, beautiful women may have been valued for their looks rather than any of their personal qualities. As a result, they may have learned to relate to others on a superficial basis and have difficulty becoming emotionally involved with their partner.

4.   Being beautiful does not increase the likelihood of marital happiness. After the novelty has worn off, you would still have disagreements with your husband about money, disciplining the kids, or whose turn it is to take out the garbage. Physical beauty certainly hasn't made divorce less likely among Hollywood actors and actresses.

5.   Frequently the husband of a beautiful woman is jealous and possessive. He assumes that other men are after her so he may become controlling and try to supervise her access to other males. Many men, although they might like to be seen with a beautiful girlfriend, would prefer to avoid these hassles when it comes to getting married.

Now, would you like to revise your fantasies? I am not suggesting that you forget about your appearance. There's nothing wrong with looking your best; just make sure that your goals are realistic. For many women, the second reason for losing weight—being healthy—is at least as important.

Thin = Healthy

I have some good news and some bad news about the health risks of being fat. The bad news you already know. Obesity is associated with coronary risk factors like hypertension and lipid problems, as well as with medical conditions such as diabetes, joint problems, gallstones, respiratory dysfunction, and the incidence of certain types of cancer.[49] The good news is that you don't need to reach your ideal weight in order to improve your health. Small weight reductions can significantly decrease your health risks! After an extensive review of medical studies, Dr. George Blackburn, an obesity expert at Harvard Medical School concluded:

> *Weight loss as low as 5% of body weight has been shown to reduce or eliminate disorders associated with obesity . . .*[50]

In one study of overweight hypertensive patients, losing as little as 11 pounds was as effective in reducing blood pressure as taking medication![51] Regardless of your ideal weight, small reductions can have a big health benefit.

Apples and Pears, Health and Beauty

When you are thinking about your health and appearance goals, remember that reaching your weight goal may not produce the perfect hour-glass shape. The distribution of fat on your body is largely inherited.[52] When you reach your goal, you will have improved your appearance and reduced your health risks even if some body parts still look fat to you.

The pattern of fat distribution on the body usually can be categorized as either an apple or a pear. If you are an apple, you tend to carry excess weight above your waist, in the chest and abdomen. In contrast, a pear accumulates fat below the waist, typically in the buttocks and thighs. These patterns are inherited. You can control the amount of fat on your body by restricting your eating and exercising, but when you have fat on your body, you won't be able to change where it is located.

Usually (but not always) women are pears and men are apples. Being a pear has some advantages. Since the fat is farther away from your heart, there are fewer health risks with pear fat than there are with apple fat. It has been estimated that women can carry up to 30 pounds below the waist without incurring any health risks. The disadvantage is that lower body fat is usually more difficult to lose than abdominal fat. If both you and your husband lose weight, he could have a flat stomach while you are still unhappy about your thighs.

Box 14. Apples vs. Pears

To get an idea of the health risks associated with your shape, measure your waist at its smallest point and your hips at its broadest. Then divide the waist measurement by the hip measurement. Health risks are greater if this ratio is more than 0.8 for females, or 1.0 for males. Keep your waist-hip ratio in mind when you set your weight reduction goals.

Like most men, I am a classic apple. If I gain any weight, it goes straight to my belly. About 10 years ago, I lost almost 20 pounds after an illness. Friends told me that I looked gaunt, and needed to put on weight. Although I was below my ideal weight, I still had my paunch. All the sit-ups I did increased the stomach muscles behind my abdominal fat but did not reduce it. While I won't deny that I would prefer to have a flat stomach, I have accepted that it is not going to happen.

Can you learn to live with cottage cheese in your bottom? According to Dr. G. Terence Wilson, a psychologist who has published many studies on eating disorders and obesity, acceptance is linked to permanent weight loss. Dr. Wilson suggests that by accepting your imperfections, you decrease the sense of deprivation that you feel when you restrict your eating.[53] Liking yourself, cottage cheese and all, will make it easier to lose weight.

Setting Your Goals

How much would you weigh if you were perfectly happy with your weight? Write this number here _____. This is your ideal weight. Now that you have written it down, you probably don't need to think about it for a while. You can set your ideal goal aside, and then work on meeting your realistic goal. When you have reached your realistic goal, you will have significantly reduced your health risks. You might be happy with the improvement in your appearance and decide to maintain your weight at this level. If not, you can come back and work on your ideal goal.

Here a few guidelines to help you set a realistic weight goal:

1. Since turning 21, what is the lowest weight you have been able to maintain for one year? Write this weight here: _____ pounds. Even if you thought you were fat when you were at this weight, would you recognize health and appearance benefits if you could get back to this weight? For most people, this would be a good realistic goal. Once you have reached this weight, you may decide that it wasn't too difficult, so you could set a new goal that is closer to your ideal weight. On

the other hand, if it took a lot of effort to get there, you could justifiably decide that this is a reasonable weight for you even if it is not your ideal weight.

2.   Are you an apple or a pear? Is your waist-to-hip ratio in the safe range? (See Box 13.) If you are a pear, your goal could make allowances for the weight you carry below the waist that is not a health risk. If you'd like, you can add several extra pounds to your realistic weight goal.

3.   Rather than have a single number for your goal, choose a 4- or 5-pound weight range as a goal. When you have reached your goal, there will still be some fluctuation in your weight. When you are at the upper end of your goal range, don't think of yourself as a failure. Instead, pay particular attention to your self-monitoring to see if there have been any subtle changes in your eating, and then make the necessary adjustments to lose a few pounds.

With these three suggestions in mind, set a tentative weight range goal and write it in here. My realistic weight goal is between _____ and _____ pounds.

Box 15.   Muscle Matters

Stepping on the scale isn't the only way to measure your progress. Actually, you are more concerned with fat on your body than with weight per se. Since muscle weighs more than fat, it is possible for you to lose fat, gain muscle, and still see the same number when you step on the scale. You can assess your progress by wearing clothes that aren't baggy or have elastic waistbands. When you put on a pair of pants that you haven't worn for a while, you'll have an idea if you're headed in the right direction.

Making Up Your Own Mind

Although you will be the only one who will decide how much you want to lose and the pace of your weight loss, you will recall from Chapter 3 that your husband has influenced your weight gain and previous attempts to diet. It's helpful if he understands your goals and hopefully agrees with them. If you are both working from the same set of assumptions, it's more likely that he will be supportive.

When you have a few minutes together, without interruptions or distractions, ask him to read the following note and then get his opinions.

A Note for Your Husband

Dear Husband,

Your wife is trying to set a realistic weight loss goal. Although height and weight charts can suggest a desirable weight for her height, these weights are not realistic for everyone. Since there are many possible reasons for weight gain (see Chapters 2 and 3), some overweight people may have more difficulty losing than others. This chapter has guidelines to help her set a goal, but it is also important for her to get your opinion before starting. She will ask you a few questions. Please try to give her honest answers, but recognize that, while your opinion is important, she will need to set a goal that is comfortable for her.

These three questions will help address some of the concerns husbands have when their wife is dieting. You can use them to discuss your goals with him.

1.   *What do you think about my current weight?* Does he think your current weight is okay, but doesn't object if you want to lose? If he thinks you look fine at your current weight, can he understand the health benefits you will gain from losing weight? If he thinks you should lose weight, does he have a specific goal in mind? How close is it to the tentative goal you have developed?

2.   *What do you think will change when I reach my goal, and how will these changes affect you?* Does he think your sex life will change? Does he have hope that there will be activities that you will be able to do together that you don't do now? Will he feel more pride when you are with him in social situations? Is he expecting that you will behave differently after you've lost weight?

3.   *Do you have any concerns about possible negative outcomes?* Is he afraid that your breasts will get smaller? Would he feel insecure, jealous, or threatened when you are thinner? Solutions for some of these problems will be discussed in later chapters, but it will be helpful if your husband is able to discuss any of these concerns now.

Terri was a 45-year-old 170-pound businesswoman who had been married to Don for 23 years. When Terri was working on her goal, she wanted input from Don. She waited until the weekend, when they had some time, and asked:

TERRI: I'd like your opinion on something. Is this a good time to ask?

DON: Let me guess. You're reading a handout from that workshop, so it must be something about your weight. Go ahead and ask.

TERRI: You're right. The second step of the program involves setting a realistic weight goal and it says that you should talk to your husband before deciding. I know you were unhappy when I got up to 180, but what do you think I should weigh?

DON: I don't know. You looked pretty hefty back then. I don't know, I guess I liked the way you looked when we got married. [She weighed 132 at their wedding but quickly gained 10 pounds.]

TERRI: That was over twenty years ago! Get real!

DON: Well, you asked. No, seriously you looked great back then, but I guess I'd be happy if you were comfortable wearing shorts and we could play tennis.

TERRI: Good. That helps. Now, I've got another question for you. If I did lose, how would that affect you?

DON: (with a tone of irritation): I already told you, I'd like it if we could play tennis.

TERRI: I don't mean to be bugging you, but I'm curious if anything about you and me would be different if I lost weight.

DON: I guess you might be willing to go on some of the easier bike rides I do. Maybe you'd be less self-conscious, and we'd have a better time at the beach. Gee, I wonder if we could take a shower together?

TERRI: Don't hold your breath, you horny old fool. Can you think of any negatives? Would anything upset you if I lost weight? Do you think I'd get more attention from the guys at work? Of course, you'd be the only one I'd shower with.

DON: That's a relief. Seriously, let me think about that one. I've gotten used to you at 170, I'm not sure if I'd have any problems if you really lost weight.

TERRI: Well, thanks for your input. Let me know if you have any more thoughts.

Don and Terri had a stable relationship and could be open with each other when talking about sensitive topics. Even so, Terri waited for a time when Don would be willing to have this talk. There were still several points in this discussion where Don started to lose patience or get irritated. Fortunately, Terri did not get defensive, or change the topic to avoid an argument (Rule 2 in Chapter 4), but instead was able to reassure him (Rule 4) and continue the discussion.

Depending upon what else is happening in your relationship, you may find it more (or less) difficult to have this discussion with your husband. If you try, and he is negative or unresponsive, don't allow your feelings to be hurt. Calm yourself (Rule 1), listen without becoming defensive (Rule 2), and try to figure out the feeling behind the response you are getting. If it seems that he is angry or frustrated, ask him for clarification, and give some thought to his answers. After you've thought about it for a few days or more, you can bring the topic up again while acknowledging his feelings that produced his negative response. If you still encounter resistance, complain but don't criticize (Rule 3) about his unwillingness to discuss your goals, let him know how important his input is to you (Rule 4), and proceed without him. The next ingredient in the Recipe, separating the heart from the stomach, will make this easier to do.

CHAPTER 7

Surgery: Separating the Heart from the Stomach

Margo was looking forward to 5:30 when Randy came home. She was upset and couldn't wait to tell him about the experience she had had at work earlier that day.

Margo was a 31-year-old office manager for a busy medical group. In the last year the office had been in constant turmoil as a result of changes brought on by managed care. Several doctors had combined their practices, which required the integration of their staffs, their medical records, billing procedures, and office routines. Margo had to oversee the whole process while being careful not to offend any of the doctors or their favorite assistants. Today had been particularly stressful because a long-simmering conflict between two of the nurses had erupted into a heated argument. Margo's efforts to mediate had not gone well and she was worried. She was concerned she might have said something that was insensitive. She needed to discuss the day's events with Randy. He would listen, make her feel better, and give her impartial feedback.

It was after 6:00 when Randy came home. He was tired, and wanted nothing more than to plop himself down on the sofa, beer in hand, and watch TV. He didn't care what was on. If the girls (they had three young daughters) were watching a repeat of an ancient sitcom, it was fine with him so long as nobody wanted anything from him. He was a nurse at the local hospital. All day long he'd been running to keep patients and doctors happy. He didn't want to listen to any more requests or demands and he was tired of smiling at people.

Can you see the collision coming? Margo will greet Randy as he walks in the door. She will launch into a detailed description of the events of the day, express her feelings, and ask his opinion about how she should handle the conflict between the nurses. Randy, trying to be polite, will nod and make an occasional perfunctory comment or grunt, but he won't become involved in Margo's dilemma or give her the type of support she is looking for. After a few minutes he will forget about being polite and focus his attention on the TV in a way that lets Margo know that he wants to end the conversation. Meanwhile Margo will become increasingly impatient as she realizes that Randy is not really paying attention to her. Her voice will get louder and take on an irritated tone. She will accuse him of not caring. Randy will be perplexed. All he wanted to do was unwind in front of the TV, yet somehow he is the bad guy involved in a fight with his wife.

After a sullenly quiet dinner, Randy will help clean up, put the kids to bed, and then resume watching TV. Margo will put a load of laundry in the washer, and try to read a magazine article. Although she has had a full dinner and isn't hungry, she will make several trips to the kitchen to snack. Still upset with Randy, she wonders if he would be more attentive if she lost weight.

Does Your Husband Ignore You?

Can you relate to Margo's dissatisfaction? Think about your marriage:

- Does your husband tune you out or withdraw when you'd like to talk with him?
- Do you think he would be more interested in you if you lost weight?
- Does he suggest or imply that he would pay more attention to you if you lost weight?
- Do you think that there would be fewer fights if you lost weight?

If you answered yes to these questions, you are a prime candidate for stomach-heart surgery. You can start by recognizing that your weight is *not* the main reason your husband is less attentive than you would like him to be. Many slender women who don't eat to console themselves complain that their husbands are distant. Even if your husband implies or says he'd give you more attention if you were thinner, it is likely that your weight is just a convenient focus for a more basic conflict revolving around the closeness vs. distance theme. This is unfortunate because when either husband or wife (or both) focus on weight, they are distracted from the real issue that divides them. They will miss the opportunity to resolve the underlying cause of the conflict. If it isn't weight, what is the real cause of the conflict in your marriage?

Closeness vs. Distance in Your Marriage

Psychologists Neil Jacobson and Andrew Christensen have been researching marital conflicts and marriage counseling for more than 20 years. They have concluded that there is one theme that underlies many different types of marital conflict. They describe the theme as:

> . . . *a struggle over the optimal level of intimacy present in the relationship. One partner, often the wife, enters therapy desiring more closeness, while the partner, often the husband, seeks to maintain an optimal (for him) amount of distance. Whether the couple is fighting about money, parenting, time spent together, or sex, the closeness-distance theme is always present.*[54]

Like many women, Margo wants more communication and closeness while Randy wants more separation. As Margo asks for closeness, Randy withdraws, leaving Margo feeling frustrated and hurt. Feeling worse, she escalates her requests for closeness. Randy experiences her persistence as an unreasonable demand, which causes him to retreat further. Usually she starts crying because of her hurt feelings, although sometimes she yells because she is angry that he is neglecting her when she needs him. Occasionally Randy is the first to get angry, yelling "leave me alone," storming out of the room, and slamming the door. Regardless of who is the first to get angry, the struggle over closeness vs. distance can be one of the most destructive patterns in a marriage

In several studies of normal-weight couples, researchers videotaped, and then rated, the couples discussing changes they would like from each other. Couples who had discussions in which the wife was demanding and the husband withdrawing were significantly less happy with their marriages at a one-year follow-up.[55] Instead of withdrawing, it was preferable when the husband argued with his wife, even though it wasn't particularly pleasant.[56]

If the conflict over closeness vs. distance is not resolved, both husband and wife will feel that their legitimate needs are being ignored by their partner. For some couples, the simmering resentment will produce frequent angry flare-ups over any trivial disagreement. For other couples, the resentment will eventually be replaced by a sense of futility. The wife will give up and seek closeness elsewhere, usually with her friends, but sometimes with a lover. Although it seems that the husband has "won" because his wife is giving him the independence he wants, after a while he may start to complain that she is cold, not very affectionate, or bitchy. Even if he does not recognize that she has withdrawn from him emotionally, he will notice that she isn't very interested in sex. Most wives find it hard to get turned on at night when their husband has been ignoring them all day.

Think about your marriage again. Do you and your husband differ in the need for closeness? Does this difference come out in arguments about a variety of topics including your weight? Have you reached the point where you are tired of asking for closeness, and look for comfort elsewhere, possibly in the refrigerator?

Food as a Consolation Prize

The unfortunate example of Maxine, a 48-year-old, 190-pound bookkeeper, is a clear example of eating being used as a substitute for closeness. Maxine was unhappily married to Dwight, a 50-year-old businessman who gambled compulsively. She described their relationship as "empty." She told me:

He brings nothing to the relationship. He is secretive and dishonest about his gambling, but I still have to take care of him and the kids. No one takes care of me; food is my consolation prize.

Maxine told me about an incident which demonstrated how this process was related to her weight. After Dwight ran up his gambling debt, she went to the card dealer and asked him not to take any post-dated checks from Dwight. The card dealer was sympathetic, understanding, and agreed to help. In the following week, Maxine had fantasies of being in love with the card dealer. She couldn't remember what he looked like, but she remembered his attention and concern for her. During that week she lost 5 pounds without any effort. When she met the card dealer again:

> The romance was gone. He smoked and he wasn't very attractive, but it showed me how much I needed someone to care about me. I never realized how much extra eating I was doing to console myself.

Although Margo's relationship wasn't as empty as Maxine's, she also used food as a consolation prize. Sometimes when she felt distance from Randy, Margo made attempts to reach out to friends for emotional support. Most of her friends had their own families and weren't always available to talk when Margo was needing companionship. Although this was not a deliberate choice on her part, she frequently found herself eating after she couldn't make contact with Randy. Even if she was able to call a friend, the urge to snack usually returned after she hung up the phone. For Margo, food became the substitute for the closeness that she couldn't get from Randy.

Stop for a moment and consider your relationship with your husband, and your relationship with food. The 3 x 5 self-monitoring cards may provide some clues. Pay particular attention to any eating that occurred after dinner. For most couples, evening provides the opportunity to be with each other. If your self-monitoring records show frequent after-dinner snacking, ask yourself, "Am I feeling lonely? Am I using food to make myself feel better?"

The Decline of Intimacy

If you have been married for several years, you may have noticed a decline in intimacy over time. One researcher found that men spent more time in intimate conversation when they were courting their future wives, but after they were married, their work or friends took precedence.[57] If you are missing the closeness that you used to have, how do you compensate for the emotional support you aren't getting from your husband? Go back to Chapter 2 and check your Depression score on the Emotional Eating Scale. If your score was above the normal-weight average (about 5), ask yourself if your depressed eating may be related to a lack of emotional support.

If you are feeling that your husband is emotionally detached and you are needing more closeness from him, why would you turn to food? Recall from Chapter 1 that the connection between food and love often starts in infancy when eating is associated with being held and comforted. This association continues throughout childhood and adolescence as parents use food for rewards, celebrations, and consolation. As an adult, when human warmth isn't available, food can be a consolation. You can use it as a substitute for the emotional support that is missing in your relationship.

Even though you are unhappy about the weight gain resulting from this type of eating, using food to compensate for the lack of closeness is not entirely irrational. Snacking doesn't completely satisfy your need for closeness, but it does have the advantage of not hurting your feelings. Food doesn't rebuff you as your husband might, so it's safer. Food won't make demands of you. You won't feel that you are indebted to the food for making you feel better. Food is also easier and more convenient than husbands or friends. Even when Randy was willing to talk, he wasn't always available at the precise moment that Margo needed him.

Food, on the other hand, is just a refrigerator door away. With microwaves, packaged convenience foods, and drive-thru windows at fast-food restaurants, there's no waiting to be consoled.

Although eating for consolation may have served a purpose for you, after heart-stomach surgery it won't be necessary. The "surgery" is performed in two steps. In the short term, you will develop methods of nurturing yourself without food. Longer term you can find the optimal closeness-distance balance so that both you and your husband get your emotional needs met, and you won't need to eat.

What to Do While Working to Increase Intimacy

Learning to nurture yourself without food is especially important if your husband is reluctant to get involved with your weight loss. If he refused to read the letter in Chapter 4 and resists your attempts to discuss your weight goals, it's unlikely that he will be interested in becoming closer. While food is the easiest, most convenient way to nurture yourself, there are other things that you can do to feel good which may be more fun, and don't add calories.

Start by thinking about things that you like to do. Be realistic. While it might be fun to take a trip to Paris or go on a shopping spree, focus on little luxuries that you don't usually allow yourself. For example, Evelyn, a woman attending one of my workshops, told me that she had the urge to snack every night. After she got her kids to bed, and tried unsuccessfully to talk to her husband, she usually sat down to read and snack. This was her time to nurture herself after a long day. Sometimes Evelyn would make a deliberate effort to resist the craving for a snack. Even though she was reading, the thought of leftovers intruded regardless of her interest in the book. I asked her about other activities she enjoyed, but couldn't find the time to do. After some thought, she remembered that she liked to soak in a warm bath. I suggested that, if her husband didn't want to talk, she should fill the tub and do her reading there. At a follow-up several weeks later she reported that the relaxation from soaking decreased the cravings so she could concentrate on her book. She felt that she was indulging herself without eating.

Barriers to Nurturing Yourself

You may feel a little funny adding self-nurturing to your daily routine especially if you think your husband will make a negative comment about it. Often, when I suggest self-nurturing activities at a workshop, some women will resist because they "don't have the time." Since many self-nurturing activities are not time-consuming (it doesn't take any longer to read a book in a bathtub than in a chair), and others that do take time are still less time-consuming than having a snack, brooding about what you ate, and then trying to lose the resulting weight. Often I suspect that time isn't the real issue. Ask yourself if you are uncomfortable with the idea that you would be deliberately doing something nice for yourself.

The idea that you spend time with the sole purpose of being nice to yourself is difficult for many women to accept. Traditionally, women have been caregivers. You may feel that it is your responsibility to take care of your husband, children, and others but it is selfish to take care of yourself.

Even if you see your primary responsibility as taking care of your family, the idea that you shouldn't nurture yourself doesn't make much sense. The next time you fly in an airplane, pay attention to what the stewardess says when demonstrating how to use the lifejacket. The announcement usually directs parents traveling with young children to put on their own lifejacket first, and then help the children with theirs. You need to take care of yourself first so that you will be available to take care of your kids. The same principle applies when you're on the ground. If you are going to be a caretaker, you will need to nurture yourself so that you will have the resources to take care of others.

A second problem for women who are struggling with their weight revolves around the idea of laziness. Do you think that anyone can be thin if only they worked hard enough ("There are no fat women, only lazy ones")? Following this distorted logic, you must be lazy since you're not thin. If you are lazy, you haven't earned the right to do anything nice for yourself. Of course, this argument ignores the inherited aspects of obesity (see Reason 1 in Chapter 2) and assumes that even when you are making progress toward your goal, you are still lazy because you haven't reached it yet. The reality is that even if you are massively obese and not dieting, your other activities should earn you the right to take a few minutes to nurture yourself.

Nurturing Activities

Regardless of whether you "don't have the time," or feel uncomfortable being nice to yourself because you should be taking care of others, or you don't deserve it because of your laziness, you still need to nurture yourself without food. If it is hard, start small. Think of something you can do for yourself that doesn't take much time. Remind yourself why you are doing whatever it is, even though you may not agree completely that you deserve to do it. If you don't have any ideas, look at the following list and see if it doesn't trigger some ideas of your own.

Sing
Listen to music
Make a collage from photos
Meditate or pray
Browse the Web
Scratch your back
Make a sketch from a photo
Give yourself a manicure
Play an instrument
Start a crafts project
Take a nap
Buy a favorite magazine and read it

Play a computer game
Refinish a piece of furniture
Do a crossword puzzle
Try new makeup
Organize a closet or desk
Play solitaire
Repot houseplants
Sew, knit, or crochet something
Practice relaxation exercises
Put a jigsaw puzzle together

Remember, the idea is to nurture yourself, not to add one more task to your day. Pick an activity that you would enjoy and makes you feel good. If organizing your closet or doing a crossword puzzle is a chore, pick something else. Also make sure that you allow yourself to feel good. Put aside your concerns for a few minutes, even if you are not entirely happy about what you did earlier in the day. It is difficult to enjoy reading in a warm bath if you are still angry with yourself for having dessert with lunch. If this is a problem, go back to Chapter 5 and practice being good to yourself.

Since it will take some time to separate the heart from the stomach, the methods presented in Box 16 will help in reducing the amount that you eat while you still have the urge to snack.

Box 16. What to Do While the Surgery Is Healing

While you are working on nurturing yourself and increasing the closeness in your marriage, you can minimize the effects of eating for consolation. First, identify when you have the greatest risk of snacking. While you may snack during the day for various reasons, eating to nurture yourself is most likely to occur at night, after dinner. What are you usually doing when you get the urge to snack? In most households, there is some type of routine. Do you sit with your husband and watch TV? Do you tidy up, and perhaps do the laundry first? Do you read, or make phone calls? Are you doing homework for a class? Once you have determined your evening routine, you will become more conscious of when you are at risk for snacking. Then you can make snacking less likely.

1. If you have a desire to eat when watching TV, do something with your hands while watching. Do needlepoint, knit, or if you're ambitious, shine your shoes or sort laundry.

2. Never snack standing up. When you are standing, you will tend to gobble your food. Instead, sit down for every bite and eat leisurely.

3. Snack in one place—the dining room, for example—away from the television. If you are watching TV, get up, get your snack, and eat it in the dining room.

4. Take your snack, cut it in half, eat the first half, and pause for one minute. At the end of the minute, you can eat the second half if you still want it. You may find that the urge has passed and you can put the remainder back in the refrigerator.

5. Try eating your snack with your nondominant

hand. This should slow the process of eating and make it easier to eat less.

Getting the Intimacy that You Need

In addition to nurturing yourself, you can help increase the intimacy in your marriage. This also is not a process that takes place overnight. It will take some time to develop a pattern of interacting which allows your needs for closeness to be met while respecting his need for independence.

According to marriage counselor John Gray, women often don't get the support they need because they don't ask for it. Maybe you assume that your husband *should* know that you're feeling lonely or unloved. After all, you are sensitive to his needs so it is only reasonable to expect that he will be sensitive to yours. He *should* care enough to stop doing whatever he is doing and pay attention to you. Alas, marriages don't always work this way. Your husband may have never learned to pick up on the cues that you give when you are needing attention from him. There is a simple solution to this problem: Ask for his attention. Although it may feel a little awkward, and you might feel rejected if he doesn't comply, don't be shy. Even if you feel guilty about gaining weight (you may still feel that you are a sinner), you are entitled to ask for attention. Make a simple, straightforward (but not demanding) request. Margo might have had more success if she had said, "I'd like to get your opinion about something that happened at work today. When you are ready, would you give me a few minutes?"

If your husband doesn't respond immediately, or fumbles around making up an excuse, don't get angry. Instead, remember the communication rules from Chapter 4. Even though you are feeling frustrated, calm yourself (Rule 1).

This is *not* the time to loudly remind him of all the nice things you have done for him. Keep in mind that your long-term goal is to increase closeness between the two of you, and even if there is no obvious sign of success this time, by remaining calm you are improving your chances for the next time. If he offers any reason for not wanting to talk, even if you think it is just a feeble excuse, listen without becoming defensive (Rule 2). It is quite likely that his excuse will help you understand his reluctance. Is he afraid that you will become emotional and he will feel uncomfortable? Maybe he thinks that you have a hidden agenda and the real reason you want to talk is to criticize him or try to change him. Or maybe it is just that he is bored with discussions of the personalities at your work and is afraid that once you start talking about them, he won't be able to escape. Once you understand his reluctance, you will be able to reassure him that it is safe to have a conversation with you when you are feeling the need to be close. For example, if Margo thought that Randy was getting tired of her discussing the people at her office, she might have prefaced her request for his attention by saying, "I know I've been talking a lot about the people at work lately, but I'd really appreciate your opinion about something that happened today. When you are ready, would you give me a few minutes?" If you think it would be helpful, ask him to read the "Note for Your Husband."

A Note for Your Husband

Dear Husband,
　　It is very common for men and women to differ in the amount of time they want to spend with each other. Usually the wife is wanting to talk and do things together, while the husband may prefer to spend

more time by himself, or with his friends. Your wife, like many women struggling with their weight, sometimes uses food to make herself feel better when she is feeling lonely. While you are not obligated to be available to talk with her whenever she wants, you may be able to help.

She is learning more effective ways of asking for attention while being sensitive to your need for some "space." Recognizing that you can politely end a conversation if it goes on too long, see if you can make yourself more available for conversation. Sometimes, a simple question like "How was your day?" and listening attentively for a few minutes is all that is needed.

You Are the Emotional Gatekeeper

Does it seem like a lot of effort to try to increase intimacy? Actually, what you have to do is not a lot of work. What makes it seem difficult is that you are risking rejection when you ask. If you are feeling unworthy because of your weight, the possibility of getting rejected is even more painful. Keep the payoff in mind: You are strengthening the relationship while decreasing your need to use food as a substitute. Also, there are fringe benefits for both you and your husband. Research has shown that intimacy is linked to happiness, contentment, and well-being. Having the opportunity to discuss upsetting information with someone who cares has been associated with improved mental and physical health.[58]

Do you think that it is unfair that you have to take the lead in increasing the intimacy in your marriage? Ideally, both of you would participate equally in an exercise that improves the relationship, yet in most marriages it is the wife who is the "emotional gatekeeper." Maybe in future generations men will be as comfortable with emotional expression as women, but right now, in your marriage, if there is going to be a change in this area, you will be the one who initiates it.

Margo persisted and was able to get more emotional support from Randy. At first, it seemed a bit artificial because the terms had to be negotiated. She would wait until he was relaxed and wasn't involved with something else, to ask for his attention. After several months they had learned to be more sensitive to each other's needs for closeness vs. distance. They recognized cues from each other, and the communication became more natural. Later on I saw Randy in my office without Margo and asked how things were going between the two of them. He was pleased with the progress she was making with her weight, but also commented that they were getting along better. He explained that she seemed less demanding so she was nicer to be around.

Using food as a consolation is a habit that may take some time to change, but with some persistence it can be done. The key is to recognize that what you are needing is nurturing, not food. Then you have a choice. You can nurture yourself, ask your husband for emotional support, or do some of both.

CHAPTER 8

Safe Sex

This chapter is not about using condoms to prevent sexually transmitted diseases. It is about feeling safe about your sexuality, regardless of your weight. Start by answering the questions below:

1. My husband gets jealous if a male compliments or pays attention to me.

Yes_____ No_____

2. When I was thinner, I got sexual attention that I did not want.

Yes_____ No_____

3. I have fantasies about having sex with someone other than my husband when I lose weight.

Yes_____ No_____

4. If I was thinner, it would be hard to cope with sexual comments and pressures from men.

Yes_____ No_____

5. If I lose weight, my husband might not be good enough for me.

Yes_____ No_____

6. I experienced sexual abuse when I was a child or was raped as an adult.

Yes_____ No_____

7. My husband is not sensitive to my sexual needs.

Yes_____ No_____

8. I remember boys in school making sexual comments about my body.

Yes_____ No_____

9. My husband pressures me to lose weight but then does things that are unhelpful.

Yes_____ No_____

10. I feel stronger when I am heavy.

Yes_____ No_____

Count the number of yeses you have checked for Questions 1, 3, 5, 7, and 9, then go back and count the yeses for Questions 2, 4, 6, 8, and 10. While this isn't a scientifically validated test, the odd items measure a tendency to use fat as a chastity belt, while the even items indicate a tendency to use fat for armor. Your scores may be a clue to help you determine if either of these patterns has contributed to your weight gain and interfered with your previous diets.

A study of 100 overweight participants in a hospital-based Optifast program found that 35 percent reported that their obesity served as a chastity belt by decreasing their husbands' jealousy or as armor by reducing their sexual fears.[59] If fat has served either as a chastity belt or as armor for you, in this chapter you will learn to deal with the underlying sexual issues that have created barriers to weight loss.

Barbara's Chastity Belt

Barbara's history illustrates fat as a chastity belt. Especially if you answered yes to three or more of the odd items, see if you can identify with Barbara's predicament.

Barbara was an outgoing, 30-year-old, stay-at-home mother who weighed 239 pounds. She was married to Joe, a quiet 31-year-old draftsman. Although she described herself as having been "bigger than the other kids" as a child, she recognized that most of her weight gain occurred after getting married. In addition to losing weight, she was seeking help with her depressed moods and her decreasing interest in sex. She wasn't sure why she didn't enjoy sex anymore. She thought that it might be because she was heavy, which made her "too tired" by the time they were ready for bed.

Barbara had several concerns about her relationship with Joe. She felt that he wasn't sensitive to her feelings, and wondered "if he finds me disgusting." Whenever she probed, Joe said he didn't object to her weight, but Joe's reassurance did not make her feel better. She also felt guilty because she was having sexual fantasies about other men. With some embarrassment, Barbara admitted that after having a sexual dream, she would wake Joe up to tell him about it. She was testing him, hoping to provoke his jealousy. This strategy didn't work. Joe seemed unconcerned when Barbara told him about her dreams.

After several sessions devoted to her weight, Barbara's eating habits didn't change. Despite her enthusiasm, and her willingness to complete the self-monitoring cards, she didn't lose any weight. While we were reviewing her self-monitoring, she casually mentioned that Joe might be "subverting" her weight program. Barbara elaborated:

Joe does all the wrong things. If I don't eat dessert, he makes a point of having some in front of me and offering me some from his plate. I feel like he is fighting me all the way, even to the point of becoming overweight himself so that he can keep me fat.

Does any of this sound familiar? Ignore the details; concentrate on the sexual jealousy and Joe's attempts to undermine Barbara's dieting. Do you see any similarities to your situation?

Men Have Sexual Insecurities Too

Recall from Chapter 7 that women usually want more closeness, while the typical male is happiest when he can maintain some independence from his wife. Barbara's attempts to make Joe jealous were intended to prod him to be closer, more romantic, and a better lover. It didn't work because Joe wasn't comfortable getting closer, and didn't know how to be more romantic or a better lover. He was in a bind. Although he may want more distance than his wife does, he felt threatened when she hinted that she might be unfaithful. Instead of getting angry or displaying jealousy, he relied on her fat to ensure that she remained faithful.

Fat as a Chastity Belt

Although neither Barbara nor Joe will discuss their concerns openly, they send thinly disguised messages to each other. By telling Joe about her sexual dreams, Barbara is letting him know of her dissatisfaction with him and her interest in other men. Instead of discussing her dissatisfaction or his own insecurities, Joe tries to ensure her faithfulness by undermining her efforts to lose weight. He believes that if Barbara is fat, he won't have any competition. This is important to him because Joe has some concerns about his own attractiveness. Also, he didn't date very much before marrying Barbara, so he is unsure about his competence as a lover. As long as Barbara stays fat, he feels safe since she should be grateful to have him for a husband. On the other hand, if Barbara did lose weight, he would have to confront his fears about his sexual performance and pay more attention to his appearance.

Barbara uses her weight as a self-imposed chastity belt. She knows that she is sexually curious but is afraid of the consequences of having an affair. Despite Joe's shortcomings, she wants to stay married to him, so she lets him disrupt her diets. Barbara believes that as long as she stays fat, she won't be tempted since no desirable male would be attracted to her. Even if she had the opportunity to have an affair, she would be too self-conscious about her body to become sexually involved.

For both Barbara and Joe, her excess weight serves a purpose. Although neither is happy, they can focus their attention on her weight and diets. This is less dangerous than dealing with the sexual dissatisfactions that they both feel. Both believe that being fat minimizes sexual urges and precludes having an affair. Both are afraid that honestly confronting the problems with their sex life would expose their respective inadequacies, and might cause the other to leave.

Fat as a Defective Chastity Belt

Most couples using fat as a chastity belt would be surprised to learn that it isn't a very effective method of ensuring fidelity, and probably isn't necessary anyway. Being fat and being faithful are two separate issues. Being fat doesn't guarantee faithfulness; being slender doesn't require infidelity. For example, Julie, a 26-year-old teacher was engaged to be married to Brian. Although they planned a wedding later that summer, she felt the need to have a "fling" with a handsome Italian she met when traveling in Europe with two of her friends. Usually she was shy, and rather modest about her 185-pound body. On vacation, all it took was a little wine and heavily accented flattery to overcome her inhibitions. After returning home, she was embarrassed as she told me about this incident and her increasingly ambivalent feelings about marrying Brian. Eventually she decided to postpone the wedding. The relevant point here is that weight and self-consciousness don't always work as a chastity belt.

What if you have been faithful to your husband but have had sexual fantasies about other men? If you suddenly lost weight, would you immediately act out your fantasies? Although fantasies can be fun, acting on them is a lot more complicated, regardless of your weight. After all, you probably know slender women who are faithful to their husbands even when they think that he's being a jerk. When you lose weight and aren't "protected" by your chastity belt, you may continue to have fantasies, but it is unlikely that you will become wildly promiscuous.

Being fat doesn't work very well as a chastity belt, but having a chastity belt can interfere with weight loss. When unresolved sexual issues in your marriage are dealt with directly, you will find it's easier to lose weight. Three common issues are sexual insecurity, sexual boredom, and difficulty communicating about sex. Let's start with sexual insecurity.

Overcoming Sexual Insecurity

For most couples, regardless of their weight, a fulfilling sexual relationship is the best insurance against an affair. When Joe and Barbara improved their sexual relationship, the chastity belt was unnecessary. Barbara started this process by improving her body image, even before she lost any weight. As she became more comfortable with her body, she was able to be more playful sexually. For example, instead of grabbing a bathrobe as soon as she finished showering, Barbara wrapped herself in a towel, and let the top slip down when Joe walked by. Joe was very happy with this new behavior and responded appropriately. He was less threatened by her attempts to lose weight as it became clear that she was still sexually interested in him. Barbara still wondered about sex with other men, but as their sexual relationship improved, it became more of an abstract curiosity instead of a frightening urge to explore.

Stop for a moment and get a mental image of your naked body. How do you feel? If you are dissatisfied, have negative thoughts ("It's gross and disgusting"), and bad feelings like shame and guilt, you will be self-conscious when making love. It's almost impossible to get totally involved in making love if you are worried about the dimples in your thighs! This is unfortunate, and may impede weight loss. One study of women in a Montreal weight loss program found that women who rated themselves as sexually attractive at the start of the program were more successful in losing weight.[60] You will benefit from working on your body image so that you can start to feel sexually desirable, even if you are many pounds away from your goal.

Although the negative thoughts interfere with sexual pleasure, and generally bring you down, you may think that hating your body is necessary to lose weight. Many dieters assume that they would lose their motivation if they didn't hate their body. This is rarely true. There are enough benefits that come with weight loss to keep you motivated without self-hatred. Besides, hating your body is a difficult habit to break. If you hate your body now, when you lose weight you'll still be dissatisfied. You won't have the fat to hate but instead you'll hate your stretch marks, the shape of your breasts, your knobby knees, or some other feature. You'll still be self-conscious when you take your clothes off, so you might as well start to get comfortable with your body now, even if you're a long way from reaching your goal.

Dr. James Rosen, a University of Vermont psychologist, developed a program to teach obese women to have a better body image and improved self-esteem. Even though they stopped hating their bodies, on average they didn't gain weight, and many reported increased feelings of being in control of their eating.[61] Having a negative body image does *not* help you to stay motivated. It just makes you feel miserable and interferes with your enjoyment of sex. Some of the methods Dr. Rosen used in his program are presented in Box 17. You can use them to feel more comfortable with your body.

Box 17. Enhancing Your Body Image

1. Recognize, from your own history and others' experiences, that actual physical appearance and body image are not always the same. Many women who aren't overweight still see themselves as fat. You may have lost weight in the past and still have a negative view of your body.

2. Remember experiences from your childhood and adolescence that may have contributed to your negative body image. Were you teased, rejected, ridiculed at sports, or criticized about your weight? Try to remember who it was who did the teasing or criticizing. When you have an image of that person, ask yourself, do you really want to let that person control how you feel about yourself?

3. Use objective descriptions of body parts (e.g., big

stomach, heavy thighs), rather than harsh judgmental terms (e.g., disgusting fat) when you discuss them. Whenever you think one of the harsh terms, correct yourself by repeating the neutral description of the same body part.

4. Learn to tolerate parts of your body that you find unattractive. Choose a trusted friend, and while clothed, direct her attention to a body part that you find particularly distressing. For example, if you hate your thighs, put on a pair of shorts and tell your friend that you are trying to become less self-conscious about your thighs. It may take a few uncomfortable minutes, but encourage your friend to look at your thighs until you can relax knowing that she is looking at them. With repetition it won't feel so awkward.

5. In public, don't try to hide body parts. For example, don't fold your arms over your stomach to hide it. Tuck your blouse in and don't be afraid to ask sales clerks for feedback when trying on clothes.

Remember that there is no reason for you to gain weight, or lose your motivation, just because you have stopped hating your body.

As you become more comfortable with your body, you will be less restrained around your husband. When you take your clothes off, it will be easier to be turned on if you aren't thinking, "I can't let him see my butt or he'll be grossed out." He will feel less threatened when he experiences your increased sexuality, and his need for your chastity belt will decrease.

The Thrill Is Gone

Can you remember a time when sex with your husband was more exciting than it is now? Even if you are completely comfortable with your body or never had a weight problem, this is a common complaint. According to Drs. Neil Jacobson and Andrew Christensen:

> . . . no matter how many manuals one uses, no matter how much variety couples inject into their sexual relationship . . . the fact remains that part of eroticism is mystery and the body of the partner becomes a bit less mysterious with each episode.[62]

If some of your concern about being faithful is a result of feeling that sex isn't as exciting as it once was, you should recognize that this may not be a result of your weight or any particular shortcoming. Having fantasies is a predictable response when real-life excitement decreases. Masters and Johnson reported that 86 percent of the women they interviewed had erotic fantasies. The most common was imagining sex with a different partner, but most fantasizers didn't feel the need to act them out in real life.[63]

If you are having sexual fantasies that don't include your husband, you don't need to feel guilty, and you certainly don't need a chastity belt to keep yourself faithful. Instead, you could try to add a little variety to your sex life. Box 18 presents a few methods that you could use. Feel free to be creative and try a few of your own.

Box 18. Getting Out of That Rut

If your sex life has become routine, boring, or nonexistent lately, don't assume that there is nothing you can do until you lose weight. Remember, a decrease in sexual interest is a common occurrence in happily married, normal-weight couples, too. Even if you are feeling self-conscious about your body, your husband is likely to appreciate your increased interest in sex before you reach your goal weight. Try the following:

1. Change the location. If you usually have sex in the bedroom, try a different room, a motel, or outside in a secluded, romantic setting.

2. Read favorite erotic passages from books or magazines to each other. Rent an erotic (not necessarily pornographic) video and watch it together.

3. Change clothing. Instead of taking your clothes off and getting into bed, pretend you're on a date and start kissing and taking each other's clothes off. If you are comfortable sharing your sexual fantasies, you can dress in the appropriate clothing and act out your fantasies with your husband.

All Action and No Talk

Another common problem is communicating about sex. Barbara and Joe are typical. They were high school sweethearts. Although she had dated other boys before she met Joe, he was her first lover. Now, 13 years later, she was curious about what she might have missed. Since having the kids, sex with Joe had become boring and infrequent. When I suggested some of the activities in Box 18, Barbara became flustered. She would feel embarrassed. She didn't know how to bring the topic up, and thought that Joe would interpret any suggestion as a criticism.

Barbara knew that Joe said he wanted sex more often, but she wasn't sure if he was dissatisfied in any other way. Unfortunately, neither Barbara nor Joe was able to discuss their feelings about sex. Apparently, this is typical of many couples. In one study,[64] both male and female participants wanted their partners to tell them what they would like sexually, yet both sexes had difficulty telling their partners what they wanted. If you are like Barbara, you are quietly waiting for your husband to figure out what to do to make you happy. As soon as he learns how to read your mind, you will have a satisfying sexual relationship!

Instead of mind reading, or gaining weight to ensure fidelity, how about increasing communication about sex? Box 19 presents a few suggestions for talking about sex.

Box 19. Talking About Sex

It helps to realize that sex can be difficult to discuss. Even people who consider themselves "swingers" frequently become embarrassed and tongue-tied when they try to talk about their sexual feelings. It's often easier to tell an explicit joke at a party than it is to tell your husband that you'd get turned on sooner if he took a shower before coming to bed. While the rules for Intergalactic Communication presented in Chapter 4 still apply, here are a few recommendations specifically for sex:

1. Keep communication short and simple. A long philosophical discourse is rarely helpful. Likewise, limit your discussion to a single sexual topic. Other topics can be discussed later.

2. If you're feeling a little awkward, it may help to ask your husband to listen for a few minutes without interruption (unless he needs clarification about something you said). Let him know that you want to hear his responses, but it would help if he listened first. Then make sure you tell him when you have finished and listen to what he has to say.

3. Communicating about sex doesn't require that you give up all your privacy. You can be honest and

straightforward without describing your previous sexual relationships or all of your fantasies.

4. Communication can be both verbal and nonverbal. You can physically guide your partner to do something, and let him know "That feels good" or "Please be a little more gentle."

5. If you have had several discussions, and you have been clear in describing your sexual preferences, but there still are no signs of change, it is likely that the difficulty is not sexual. Maybe there are control issues or your husband is angry about something else. This should be explored at a convenient time, when you're not in bed.

Unlocking the Chastity Belt

Let's assume that you don't need excess fat tissue to keep your libidinous urges in check. How are you going to persuade your husband that you are trustworthy? He will need to know that, even when you shed many of those excess pounds, you will still prefer to be with him. Even if you haven't lost much weight yet, as you become comfortable with your body, you can let him know that you are sexually interested in him. Would he feel reassured if you took the lead in initiating sex, or would that be threatening? Would he enjoy it if you were more playful? You could experiment and see what type of response you get, and then use the guidelines in Box 19 to discuss what happened. Remember that being fat and being faithful are two separate decisions. When both you and your husband see weight and sex as independent of each other, weight loss can proceed with fewer disruptions.

Kathy's Armor

Kathy was an attractive, 160-pound, 26-year-old, red-headed graduate student. She had an on-and-off relationship with Curt, who was also a 26-year-old part-time graduate student. Although the relationship had continued for five years, Kathy didn't see any future for herself with Curt. She thought that he was unmotivated and she didn't approve of his daily marijuana use. She told me that she knew she "should get on with her life" but made no serious attempts to date other men, even during the periods when she wasn't involved with Curt. When other men showed interest in her, she thought about going out with them, but usually decided that she would need to lose weight first.

Kathy was heavy when she met Curt, and although she had made several unsuccessful attempts to diet, her weight had stayed fairly constant. Curt didn't seem to care about Kathy's weight but he made an occasional sarcastic comment if she was eating candy or dessert.

As we retraced her history, Kathy noted that she wasn't overweight as a child. Although she was shy, she was popular in high school, a good student, and had a date or social activity almost every weekend. In her junior year, she went out with an older boy who pressured her to have sex with him. She was fuzzy describing the details but it sounded like date rape. Judging from her discomfort as she described this episode, Kathy still felt some guilt and shame. Afterward Kathy became more cautious in her interactions with men and started to gain weight. She could verbalize her fears although she hadn't quite made the connection to the date rape:

> *I know that I should break up with Curt, lose weight, and date other guys, but every time we break up I get scared if*

someone shows any interest in me. I don't know what's going to happen. I always end up back with Curt. It's just easier. I feel safer.

Kathy's problem is different from Barbara's. Barbara's husband was jealous and went to great lengths to keep her fat. In contrast, Curt does not undermine Kathy's diets and seems unconcerned about her weight. Even though Curt is not a threat, Kathy is afraid of losing weight. Without the weight, she would feel defenseless against unwanted sexual advances. For Barbara, fat serves as a chastity belt, while for Kathy, it is protective armor.

Fat as Armor

Have you ever felt safer because you were heavy? When you lose weight, do you feel scared or vulnerable? Unfortunately many women like Kathy had frightening sexual experiences when they were thinner. As a result, they find comfort, security, protection, and sometimes power when they are fat. The added weight serves as armor to protect against physical and emotional sexual assaults. Several recent studies have shown that using fat as armor is especially common among women who were abused as children or raped as adults. For example, Dr. Vincent Felitti reviewed the medical records of adults who had a routine physical exam at a medical clinic. One hundred thirty-one answered yes to the question, "Have you ever been raped or sexually molested?" On average, the sexual abuse had occurred more than 30 years earlier, and most of the patients had not discussed it before participating in the study. Sixty percent of the abused patients were 50 pounds or more overweight, and 25 percent were more than 100 pounds overweight. The frequency of obesity was much lower for patients who had not experienced sexual traumas.[65]

A history of sexual abuse also makes treatment more difficult. Researchers at Brown University School of Medicine found that obese women who had been abused didn't lose as much weight as the other participants in a hospital weight loss program. The abused women also gave up more often and had more difficulty with emotional eating. The authors think that weight loss is uncomfortable because the abused women have less "protection," which makes them feel more vulnerable to future abuse.[66]

Think about your history. Do you recall instances of molestation or rape? Even if it happened many years ago, or if there was no physical force, just verbal pressure, the horrible feeling of not being able to control your involvement in sex may have contributed to your weight. If you are not sure, ask yourself if there was a time when you experienced a rapid weight gain. Dr. Felitti found that often sudden weight gains followed sexual abuse,[67] so this could be a clue.

Even if you are pretty sure that you weren't abused, you may still need the armor that fat provides. Especially if you were overweight in childhood or adolescence, you might not have had enough experience with boys to have learned to comfortably reject their demands. Without this experience, interacting with men when there is even a hint of flirtation may make you feel vulnerable. Now review your responses to questions 2, 4, 6, 8, and 10 at the beginning of this chapter. Do you see any patterns? Are you using your weight as armor?

How Fat Becomes Armor

In many Middle Eastern countries, traditional Moslem women wear a veil when they leave their homes. Generally men respect the veil and reserve their stares and comments for nonveiled women. The veil provides the same kind of armor as fat does in Western society. Fat lets men know that you are off-limits for any kind of sexual attention. As a result, you can be more comfortable and feel safer when you are around men.

Fat can serve as armor because in our culture it is considered unattractive so few men would be interested in having sex with a fat woman. It is also assumed that anyone can lose as much weight as they would like, so a woman who has not lost weight to make herself more desirable must be asexual. These assumptions are clearly wrong. Many overweight women (Julie, for example) are sexually active, and the linkage between a slender body and sexual desirability is a recent cultural phenomenon that may not be terribly important when a man and a woman are together. As Betty, a 45-year-old woman, told me:

> *Mel [her husband] likes movies where skinny actresses take their clothes off, and he is always looking around when we're at the beach, but when the two of us are alone in the bedroom, I'm the one that he looks at and gets turned on by.*

How does fat become armor? Think about your experiences in elementary and junior high school. From puberty on, female bodies are the object of sexual attention. You can probably remember comments when you were in school about your developing breasts. Whether the comments were made by boys or girls, were flattering or derogatory, they made you feel uncomfortable and self-conscious. When you gain weight, the various features of your body are less well defined. You will still hear comments about your body. The comments are likely to be unpleasant or downright insulting, but you won't feel sexually threatened by them. The armor is protecting you and becomes difficult to give up.

Debbie, a 35-year-old teacher, lost 30 pounds and has started working out at a gym. She described her ambivalent feelings about giving up her armor:

> *I'm starting to really see the definition in my arms and legs. Obviously a lot of other people notice too. I've met more people, mostly men, at the gym in the past two or three months than I have in the past two years! One guy even asked me out on a date! I'm getting a lot more attention than I used to. It feels good, but I'm not sure I like it. It was like I wasn't even there before; no one noticed me. Now, I know some people take notice. It's a strange feeling. It takes getting used to. It's kind of uncomfortable.*

Even though there weren't any obviously sexual or threatening comments, Debbie felt vulnerable when men noticed her body. Without support and encouragement, it would have been easy for her to avoid the gym and regain her armor.

Feeling Safe Without Armor

If you think that you acquired your armor in response to sexual abuse, it may be helpful to find a psychologist or counselor who can help you understand your feelings about what happened to you. With help, many women are able to overcome the sense of helplessness that frequently results from sexual abuse. For example, after Kathy recognized what had happened to her, we spent some time working through her feelings about it. She became more self-confident, gradually lost weight, and eventually ended the relationship with Curt.

As you lose weight, you may get more attention, but

you're not as vulnerable as you were when you were younger. In Chapter 9 you will become more confident in your ability to politely, but firmly, say no to unreasonable requests. You will not need your excess weight for armor.

CHAPTER 9

Don't Swallow It or Spit It Out—Chew on It

Do you get angry, mad, or indignant? How about irritated, annoyed, or pissed off? The English language has dozens of words and expressions that describe angry feelings. I don't know if it's a coincidence, but many of them, like "fed up" or "spit it out," seem to relate to eating. You may also notice a connection between your eating and anger. In this chapter you will understand your angry feelings, and how they relate to your eating. To get started, check your Anger and Frustration score on the Emotional Eating Scale in Chapter 2, then we can develop methods for dealing with these feelings without eating.

Remember Rita and Tom, the unhappy couple who were described in Chapter 3? His controlling behaviors made Rita angry so she ate fattening foods to get back at him. Eventually, she got tired of his "It's my way or the highway" edicts and divorced him. When I first saw Rita, she attributed her weight gain to her pregnancies. When we explored her relationship with Tom and her eating habits more closely, a pattern emerged. See if you recognize any similarities to your own experience.

Rita married Tom as soon as she graduated from high school, promptly had two children, and became a full-time mom. Since she never had the opportunity to establish an identity as an independent, self-sufficient adult, she allowed Tom to take control. He decided which church they would join, where they went on vacation, what her household responsibilities would be, and so on. During the early years of the marriage, Rita focused on being a mom and willingly accepted his control of the other areas in her life. As her girls got older, she had more contact with other women her age and started feeling restless. Tom would object whenever Rita proposed any change in their well-ordered life. He simply forbade her to get a job or take a class at the community college.

One morning, as Tom was leaving for work, Rita mentioned that she had made plans to have dinner with a few of her friends. He went ballistic, yelled that she couldn't go, slammed the door, and drove off. Rita was upset. She felt agitated; an inner turmoil prevented her from getting on with the day's activities. As she got the girls ready for school, she stopped several times to snack. Eating might soothe the turmoil and make the bad feelings go away.

During the years between having the girls and her divorce, this scenario was repeated many times with the predictable weight gain ensuing. At first Tom didn't object. Rita was a good cook and he had put on a few pounds himself. As she continued to gain weight, her eating became more of an issue. He would make unflattering comments about her body when his friends came over and pointedly reminded her about her diet whenever she was eating high-calorie food. Rita's eating became another issue for Tom to control. Looking back, Rita told me about her anger:

I don't remember being mad very often. I think I was eating to stuff down my angry feelings. Once in a while, I'd explode and yell and slam doors, but I felt so bad afterwards, like I'd been a real bitch. Later Tom would remind me how irrational I was, and I knew that I shouldn't have carried on like that, so maybe he was right. The next time, I'd try not to explode, I'd have something to eat. Eventually, when he started nagging me about my weight, I'd deliberately eat to piss him off, even if he wasn't there.

Although she didn't recognize it at the time, Rita was angry but didn't think that she should be. Even if she had recognized her anger, and accepted it as a legitimate feeling, she did not know how to express it in a productive manner. As a girl, she never saw women expressing appropriate anger. Her mother would sulk for days on end but didn't get noticeably angry. When Rita got angry, she was admonished to behave. Now as an adult, she didn't recognize when she was angry. She used food to help suppress her anger.

Expressing vs. Suppressing Anger

One group of researchers looked at articles in psychology journals during a seven-year period and found more than 7,000 articles on anxiety, 15,000 on depression, but only 704 on anger.[68] Since we don't know very much about anger, it's not surprising that experts offer conflicting advice. You've probably read articles encouraging you to express your anger. This is difficult if, like Rita, you are a traditional female who has learned to suppress anger at all costs. Psychologist Harriet Goldhor Lerner describes this pattern as the "nice lady syndrome."[69] There are at least three problems with being a "nice lady":

1.   If you always suppress your anger, people may take advantage of you and you won't get your needs met.

2.   Suppressing anger may increase your risk of medical difficulties like hypertension, heart problems, and possibly cancer.[70]

3.   Suppressed anger may build up until it erupts like a volcano.

The obvious conclusion is to let it all hang out. When you feel anger, you should immediately express it. According to one psychiatrist, expressing anger produces "increased self-esteem and the feel of real peace with one's self and others."[71] This is the "catharsis" that keeps you healthy and brings a peaceful end to the angry episode. So, the next time someone is unfair to you, just let them have it, right? It's not that simple. Expressing your anger can be a mixed blessing. Consider the following:

1.   Modern life presents a continuing stream of irritants. It's not fair that the driver in front of you cut you off, the telephone salesperson interrupted your dinner, or your neighbor's dog pooped on your driveway. If you express every angry feeling, your life will become a series of rage episodes with only brief interruptions.

2.   The relationship between anger and health is complicated. There is evidence indicating that expressing anger can have negative health consequences.[72]

3.   Anger can feed on itself so that once you are angry, it is easier for you to become angered again. Instead of experiencing a period of tranquillity, you may have another burst of anger, and then feel guilty because you've been a "bitch." Also, consider the model you are giving your children. Do you want to raise angry kids?

Diane was an example of a woman who rarely suppressed her anger. She was referred to me by her physician, who had unsuccessfully tried several antidepressants to help her control her temper. At 46, she had been married twice before and her current marriage was shaky. In the first few sessions she described the conflicts in her relationships with her current and past husbands, her adult children, and various coworkers and neighbors. She became quite heated as she discussed all the injustices she had suffered. I started to wonder how long it would be before I did something that would make her angry with me! Fortunately, as she became comfortable, she was able to focus on her thoughts that made her angry, rather than continuing to discuss everyone else's shortcomings.

Where Anger Comes From

When you think about things that make you angry, you'll find a common theme that runs through them. It is the idea of unfairness. Like most emotions, anger starts with an interaction with another person. Something that the person has done has caused you unnecessary pain or discomfort. Even if it's something trivial, like a phone call interrupting your dinner, you think that it's unfair, that he or she "should have known better." If the pain or discomfort is more serious, you may continue to think about it. As you rehash the episode in your mind, your body may become aroused. With each repetition, the anger grows. Soon you feel your heart pumping, your face is flushed, and your muscles tighten. If this arousal continues, you will feel uncomfortable until you can release the tension by shouting, hitting, throwing, or breaking something. When the tension is discharged, you feel better for a few minutes, but then you start to feel guilty. Looking back, your angry outburst reminds you of a child's temper tantrums. You feel foolish. You vow never to lose your temper again. The next time someone does something that causes you pain or discomfort, you try to suppress your anger and eat.

What a dilemma. Should you be a "nice lady" like Rita and suppress your anger, even if you have to eat to do it, or do you let yourself be a "bitch" like Diane and make everyone else, and ultimately yourself, unhappy? Fortunately, you have a third choice. Instead of suppressing or expressing anger, you can choose to be annoyed.[73]

Annoyance vs. Anger

When you are annoyed, you don't feel your heart pumping and you aren't seething. When you are annoyed, you can think rationally and express yourself assertively so that you are treated better the next time. When you are annoyed, you don't try to forget about it like a "nice lady." You know that you have been wronged, but you can take a more philosophical view of it. You examine the incident in context and recognize how you have been hurt. Since you don't feel the physical arousal of anger, you don't need to do anything dramatic to make yourself feel better or eat to soothe yourself after an outburst.

How to Be Annoyed

If you have spent years trying to suppress your anger, you never learned to be annoyed. You may be afraid that allowing yourself to be annoyed will cause an eruption of the angry volcano that has been building just below your nice exterior. Alternatively, if you're in the habit of flying off the handle, you may think that your anger is inevitable

—there is nothing you can do about it. The reality is that you can learn to be annoyed instead. Here are five rules to help:

Rule 1: Watch Your Language

When confronted with an irritant, what do you say? Instead of "he pissed me off," "I can't stand it," or "that bugs me," substitute less forceful terms. Phrases like "that's irritating" or "I don't like it" express your annoyance without setting you up for an angry outburst.

Rule 2: Check Your Expectations

Do you use the words "should" or "must" frequently? Statements like "He should know better" suggest that you have well-defined expectations of others (and probably yourself). When these expectations aren't met, you're likely to become angry. Instead, think in terms of preferences. Instead of "He shouldn't have done that," substitute "I wish he was more thoughtful."

Rule 3: Avoid Mind Reading

When someone does something distressing, the temptation is to assume that they are purposely trying to harm you, and then to get angry. Although the person may have harmed you, unless you are a mind reader, it's unlikely that you know why they did it. Thoughtlessness, ignorance, clumsiness can result in hurtful behaviors which are annoying. Reserve your anger for situations where you definitely know (not when you think) that the other person intended to harm you.

Rule 4: Unfairness Happens

It may not be fair that it rained the last three times you had a picnic while your neighbor has sunshine for hers. When you read the newspaper, many of the stories seem unfair. Keep in mind that you cannot correct all the injustices in the world. When you can help, by all means do so, but just getting angry doesn't accomplish anything.

Rule 5: Accept Human Fallibility

The world is filled with thoroughly fallible human beings. Even otherwise admirable people—you and I, for example—will occasionally bring discomfort to others. Sometimes it is possible to understand why a person behaves in a way that you find annoying. When you understand, the behavior is still annoying, but it will have less of an effect on you.

What to Do with Your Annoyance

Once you learn to be annoyed, rather than suppressing or expressing anger, what do you do with your annoyance? You have three choices. Remember that you aren't seething and your heart is not pumping furiously, so you can think rationally and choose the option that makes the most sense.

1. You can end the interaction. Especially if you are talking to a person that you don't know and won't talk to again—a telephone salesperson, for example—just say "I'm not interested" or "I gotta go now" and hang up. When someone intrudes on your day with an annoying call, you are not obligated to provide a detailed explanation for your lack of interest in their

conversation. If they refuse to accept your simple statement, hang up, close the door, leave the room, or do whatever else it takes to end the interaction without any further discussion. If you are having an annoying conversation with a person who is more significant in your life—your mother or your husband, for example—you may need a more detailed explanation before ending the interaction, but you are still entitled to end it. For example, you could say, "I don't want to talk about this now" or "I'll talk with you later, when you have calmed down," and then hang up, close the door, or leave the room.

2. You can do nothing. Remember, you are not angry so accepting annoyance is not suppressing anything. If the annoyance was a one-time event, especially if it was accidental, you don't have to do anything in response. After a few minutes the annoyed feeling will go away and you can get on with the rest of your day.

3. You can try to change the other person's behavior. This is the most complicated response to annoyance. While there is no guarantee that you will be successful, if the annoying behavior is likely to be repeated, it is worth a try. Even if the behavior doesn't change, you will feel better having tried.

How to Change Annoying Behavior

Kelly was a 28-year-old nurse, married to David, a 29-year-old engineer. They had been married six years but didn't have any children primarily because David felt that he was "too selfish" to be a parent. Although David was much less controlling than Tom (Rita's husband), Kelly, like Rita, was a "nice lady" who ate to stuff her bad feelings. In one session we were reviewing her 3 x 5 self-monitoring records. I asked her what had been going on before she had an 8:30 P.M. "snack" consisting of M&M's, three oatmeal cookies, a piece of German chocolate cake, and an orange cupcake. When we traced the evening's events, there was nothing out of the ordinary until we got back to 5:30 in the afternoon.

When David came home from work, Kelly showed him the new walking shoes she had bought on sale. Instead of sharing her enthusiasm, David responded sarcastically. Kelly explained:

KELLY:	I was so pleased with myself. I've been walking a lot so I wanted to get a decent pair of shoes. I waited until they went on sale but he still wasn't happy.
DR. A:	What did he say?
KELLY:	He told me that I was wasting money, that we needed to save for a house. The usual speech I get when I buy anything. He doesn't yell or anything, he just makes me feel stupid and guilty.
DR. A:	You just feel stupid and guilty?
KELLY:	Yeah. I don't say anything, but I keep thinking about what he said and how unfair it is. When *he* buys something, I don't give *him* a hard time.
DR. A:	It sounds like you get really annoyed when David is being unfair. What do you do when this happens?
KELLY (pause):	I don't know . . . Nothing, I guess . . . What can I do? I don't want to be a bitch.
DR. A:	Let me see if I've got this right. When David treats you unfairly, instead of getting annoyed and letting him know why you are annoyed, and what you want him to do differently, you just sit there

KELLY:

> quietly, have angry thoughts, and then go eat.
>
> Oh. Yeah. I never thought of it like that.

Kelly went on to give me other examples and then we discussed the difference between anger and annoyance. Her expectations of David and her understanding of his motivations seemed reasonable. After more discussion, she concluded that it was okay for her to express her annoyance with David. Since she wanted to improve their relationship, she would try to change his annoying behavior. I suggested that she:

- Define the specific annoying behavior.
- Briefly describe her feelings and why changing the behavior is important.
- Ask for a specific change in behavior.
- Show appreciation for efforts to change annoying behavior.

Kelly decided that she would like to tell David:

Yesterday you criticized me when I told you about the walking shoes I bought. I feel annoyed and hurt because I want to save as much as you do, but I really needed the shoes, and I waited until they were on sale to buy them. In the future, please don't criticize my spending until you know all the details.

Although Kelly thought that this was a reasonable request, she wasn't sure she would be comfortable saying this to David. I had her practice saying it to me until she could do it easily, and then tell him that evening.

David did not apologize profusely, and promise never to criticize again, but he did listen respectfully. He admitted that it was not unreasonable for Kelly to have a new pair of shoes. She was pleased and gave him a hug.

Box 20. The Fine Art of Saying No

Many women have difficulty saying no without feeling guilty, apologizing profusely, and offering lengthy explanations. Psychologists Melanie Katzman, Lillie Weiss, and Sharlene Wolchik suggest that weight-conscious women have extra difficulties saying no because they are afraid that they might hurt someone's feelings, the other person might not like them, or that by refusing a request, they might appear to be incompetent.[74] Recognize that regardless of other people's feelings, or their perceptions of you, you have the right to refuse their requests. Besides, even if you don't say no, and end up doing something you don't want to do, they still might not like you or think that you are incompetent. Saying no is easiest when you:

1. Use short, simple, direct statements like, "I'm not having dessert tonight, thank you" without giving lengthy explanations or rationales.

2. Focus exclusively on the request being made of you. Don't let the other person manipulate you with guilt, threats, or pleading.

3. If the other person is rude enough to continue making the same request repeatedly, you can respond like a broken record, repeating the same short refusal after each request. You need not worry about being rude when you are a broken record. Judith Martin, the etiquette columnist known as "Miss Manners," advised a reader who, despite her refusals, was repeatedly urged to eat dessert:

Saying "No, thank you" does work. But like child-rearing, it may have to be repeated for 20 years before it gets through . . . Miss Manners is afraid you just have to keep repeating your polite refusal.

Your failure to engage in a conversation about the matter should eventually bore even the most persistent person.[75]

Don't Swallow Your Pride When You Are Fed Up

Review your self-monitoring cards. Even if you haven't been entirely reliable in your record keeping, you may find instances where you ate in order to "stuff" your angry feelings, or to soothe yourself after you exploded and "spit it all out." If you are not sure, find an episode of unnecessary eating (you ate even though you weren't hungry and you didn't particularly enjoy the food) and try to remember what was happening before you started to eat. What were you doing? Who was with you? What did they say or do? Try to visualize the scene. When you have a clear picture, think if anyone was treating you unfairly. Then answer the following questions:

1. Name of the person treating you unfairly. ____
2. What he or she was doing. _____

_____

3. Review Rules 1–5 and decide if you were annoyed: Yes_____ No_____
4. If you were annoyed, it is too late to end the interaction but you can still choose to: (a) do nothing; or if the annoying behavior is likely to occur again: (b) try to change the annoying behavior. (Choose and underline one.)
5. If you are going to try to change the annoying behavior, write a specific description of the behavior to be changed. _____

_____

6. Briefly describe your feelings when the behavior occurs and why change is important.

_____

_____

7. The specific change in behavior you would like is: _____

8. You will show appreciation for attempts to change behavior by:_____

_____

When you have answered these eight questions, you will have a plan for dealing with being annoyed without eating. If you are afraid that you won't be able to carry out the plan, practice. When you are alone, read your answers to 5, 6, and 7 out loud so you can hear how they sound. If necessary, you can make minor modifications as long as they don't undermine the importance of what you are saying. Practice again, this time in front of a mirror. Notice your facial expression and body language as you repeat your statements. Try to maintain eye contact (look at yourself in the mirror while talking), and keep an erect posture. Repeat several times until you can make the statements easily. Make sure you don't preface your statements with apologies like "I'm sorry" and don't offer additional lengthy explanations for the request you are making.

Are You Annoying?

In this chapter, we have been focusing on your feelings of annoyance when other people treat you unfairly. Now it's time to turn things around and consider when you are being annoying. Don't get defensive. Remember: nobody's perfect; we're all fallible human beings (see Rule 5). Even if you are a "nice lady" who goes to great lengths to avoid making other people unhappy, the reality is that sooner or later you will miscalculate and be annoying.

What does your husband do when you are being annoying? Does he swallow his anger or spit it out? Commonly accepted wisdom is that men get angry and let it out while women are "nice ladies" and suppress angry feelings. Research shows that this is not true. Men and women are more similar than different in dealing with anger. For example, men and women may become angry about different things,[76] and women cry when they are angry more often than men do,[77] but a man can express his anger and be just as "bitchy" as a woman, or suppress it and be a "nice gentleman." For example, when Rita's husband, Tom, would yell, "It's my way or the highway," he would qualify as a "super bitch." On the other hand, David made occasional sarcastic comments but rarely expressed his anger directly.

Unless he already knows how to be annoyed, your husband could benefit from reading this chapter. Even if he did not show any interest in helping you when you were reading Chapter 4, he might have more interest in reading a chapter that will help decrease your behaviors which he finds annoying.

Erase your answers to Questions 1–8 and ask your husband if he would like to read a short section on changing your annoying behaviors. Show him the "Note for Your Husband", and encourage him to answer the questions. If he is not interested, wait until he is annoyed with something you do. If he gets angry, allow him to cool off first, and ask again if he would like to help you to change the annoying behavior. Then give him the chapter to read.

A Note for Your Husband

Dear Husband,

What do you do when your wife makes you angry? Would you like to learn an effective approach to changing those irritating behaviors? The focus of this chapter has been on her angry feelings and how they are related to eating. She is learning a constructive way of letting others know when she is annoyed, and asking for specific changes in behavior. This approach should also be useful when you want her to change an annoying behavior. You can start by reading the chapter, and answering the eight questions. While you will still have disagreements, there won't be angry outbursts when you both use these methods.

Frequent expressions of anger from either you or your husband can have a corrosive effect on a marriage. Avoidance of all angry feelings may preserve peace but it will increase the emotional distance between you. Learning to express and resolve legitimate differences, even when there are bad feelings, is much healthier for both your marriage and your weight.

CHAPTER 10

Ending Food Fights

In Chapter 3 we met Sarah, the 37-year-old mother who had gained 50 pounds in 11 years of marriage. Her husband, Jerry, kept giving her mixed messages about her weight. While he pressured her to lose weight, he "forgot" whenever she needed his help, complained about the cost of her diet program, and acted hurt when she went walking with her friend. This was not a deliberate effort to make Sarah fat. Instead it was a gradually evolving pattern which required her to be overweight in order to maintain the equilibrium in the marriage.

Although it may not be obvious, unless you are a newly-wed, it is likely that your weight has become part of the equilibrium in your marriage. To proceed with A Recipe for Losing Weight and Improving Your Relationship, you will identify the role weight may play in the marital balance, and then disengage weight so that you can lose weight without causing conflict in your marriage. Let's start with a look at the rules in your marriage.

The Rules of Marriage

Every group that you belong to, whether it is large or small, a casual circle of friends, or a formal organization, has rules which influence your behavior. For example, if you are an American, it's likely that you'll have picnics and watch fireworks on the Fourth of July. If you belong to the Soroptomists, you will go to luncheons and listen to speakers. Even if the rules aren't explicitly stated, they still influence your behavior. It is unlikely that you would sing "Jingle Bells" and exchange gifts on July Fourth. It's not against the law, and no one ever told you not to sing "Jingle Bells" in July; you just don't do it. Smaller groups, the group of you and your husband, for example, also develop unstated rules and expectations.

Many marital rules revolve around the assignment of responsibilities. In a traditional marriage, the husband went to work while the wife stayed home and took care of the kids and the home, but even in less traditional marriages, there are still rules. Maybe both partners have jobs but he cooks and she does the yardwork.

Some rules don't pertain to specific responsibilities but are general expectations for behavior. For example, it may be assumed that when the husband makes a decision, it will be rational, based on a logical analysis of the alternatives, while the wife will be more emotional and impulsive. Alternatively, he could be the unrealistic dreamer with his head in the clouds, while she is the practical one who takes care of business. I am not suggesting that any of these rules are good or bad, fair or unfair, but rather that all marriages have rules. Life would get very complicated if you had to negotiate each chore every day. Instead of daily chaos, over time both partners develop expectations and a stable pattern of interacting develops. Unfortunately, the stable pattern, or equilibrium, frequently includes the wife's extra weight.

The Rules for Overweight Wives

In your marriage, especially if your husband is slender, there are rules that deal with your weight. For most couples, it is assumed that she will be concerned about her weight, and make at least occasional efforts to reduce. Even if your husband says he doesn't care about your weight, he would have an opinion if he came home and found you finishing a half gallon of ice cream. In many marriages the rules specify what the overweight wife should eat, shouldn't eat, what she should wear (no bikinis), what she should do (exercise), shouldn't do (anything that draws attention to her body), and how she should feel about her body (ashamed). Think about your own marriage. Aside from your eating, have any rules developed because of your weight?

Several prominent family therapists have suggested that, as long as both husband and wife are focused on the rules about her weight, they maintain peace by avoiding other issues that separate them.[78] If the wife starts to lose weight, the peace is threatened. Often the husband will interfere with her diet so that they don't have to confront other issues. In a survey of over 200 physicians treating obesity, 90 percent reported cases in which the husband sabotaged his wife's weight loss efforts.[79] For example, Jerry used Sarah's weight to avoid taking responsibility for coming home late and to "win" arguments with her. Sarah, feeling bad about her weight, didn't press the issue when she was unhappy about something Jerry had done. As long as she stayed fat, they could minimize conflict. When Sarah started losing weight, the equilibrium was upset since Jerry would become more accountable for his behavior. Sarah would have a stronger position in any argument. Sensing the changes that were occurring with her weight loss, Jerry brought home ice cream and complained when she went walking. Although he didn't seem to be aware of his motivations, he was trying to undermine her diet so that she would gain weight and restore the balance in their relationship.

Some husbands will try to restore equilibrium by a broader-based attack on their wives. Instead of undermining her diet, they attempt to undermine her self-esteem. For example, Kristen lost 65 pounds and started a new job. Although her husband seemed supportive at first, he quickly tried to restore the equilibrium that had been upset by her weight loss and new job.

He tells me how much he likes the new, sexy me without all the weight, but then he seems to be playing on my insecurities and I feel awful. He'll go on for hours telling me all the mistakes I make and how thoughtless and insensitive I am, then say something like, "But I still love you," as if he is the only one in the world who ever would. It makes me feel like shit.

Box 21. Judge Not

Recall from Chapter 5 that being overweight is often seen as a visible sign of immorality. If you accept this view, then it is reasonable for people who are "morally superior" to comment about your eating "for your own good." This is the implicit rationale behind many of the tactics that husbands use to maintain the equilibrium in their marriages. If you have given up yo-yos, and changed your thinking about dieting (Chapter 5), you know that you are not immoral because of your weight. You are fully capable of making your own decisions about eating. There is no need for others to intervene unless you want them to. Help your husband and other family members to recognize this by the following:

1. Don't sneak food. When you try to hide your eating, you imply that you are doing something bad,

and if he catches you, he has the right to admonish you for it.

2. Don't make excuses for your food choices. Everyone, including your husband, occasionally slips up. If you act ashamed or try to justify your eating, you are again accepting that he should be the judge of your behavior.

3. Don't lie about your weight. If you discuss your weight with your husband, tell him exactly what the scale says, even when the news isn't good.

Finding the Equilibrium in Your Marriage

Think about your own marriage. Focus on the last disagreement you had with your husband. Visualize what started the disagreement, what you said, what he said, and how it ended. Now, ask yourself:

1. Did your weight or eating become part of the discussion even though it was not the original topic?

2. Do you think the main issue being discussed was lost as the focus shifted to your weight or eating?

3. Did the discussion end with a statement about your weight or eating?

4. Have you ever been afraid to bring up a controversial topic because you thought it would turn into a discussion of your weight or eating?

If you answered yes to any of these questions, it is likely that your weight has become part of the equilibrium in your marriage. If you think about equilibrium as a balance scale, your weight is on one side, but what is on your husband's side of the scale? What does he gain when you are overweight? What would he have to change if you lost weight? The chart below shows how negative characteristics of the husband can be "balanced" by having an overweight wife:

Husband's Characteristics	How His Wife's Weight Creates Balance
He is overweight.	As long as his wife is overweight, he doesn't need to make any serious effort to lose weight. If she loses weight, he feels implicit pressure to do the same.
He has addictive behaviors.	She is in no position to criticize his smoking, drinking, gambling, or drug use as long as she is fat. When she loses weight, his behavior may come under closer scrutiny.
He feels he has lost power or control.	When she is fat, she is stigmatized so she has less power and is easier to control.
He is disappointed in himself or feels like a failure.	If she can lose weight, he should be able to do whatever it takes to be more successful.
He is worried about his declining interest in sex.	As long as she is fat, he can blame her body for his lack of interest. When she loses weight, he is confronted with his problem.
He is angry.	Even if the anger has nothing to do with his wife, her eating and weight provide a target for the anger. When she loses the weight, he loses the justification for his anger.

Do you recognize any of these patterns in your marriage? Now let's see exactly what happens when you upset the balance by losing weight.

Breaking the Rules

If you break the rules in a marriage, even though the rules were never explicitly stated, you will be pressured to conform. For example, what would happen if you sang "Jingle Bells" in July? At the very least, your husband would ask why you are doing it. Now how would he respond if you violated any of the rules that deal with your weight? If your weight has been part of the equilibrium for several years or more, and you start to lose, you can expect turmoil. Sandy and Steve provide an example of this process.

Sandy was a tall, 185-pound, 29-year-old mother of a 2-year-old girl. She had worked as a dental assistant for six years, but at the time she was back in school studying marketing. Her husband, Steve, a 30-year-old pharmacist, was unhappy working for his father in the family-owned drugstore. At our first session, Sandy told me:

Steve always said he wanted me to lose weight but it's never been a big problem until I actually started to lose a few months ago. Now it's always an issue.

She went on to describe some of the fights they'd had about her weight:

He's a dirty fighter. He goes for my weak spots. He makes nasty comments about my butt. We're going to Hawaii next month. I'm dreading the comments he's going to make when I wear a bathing suit. A couple of days ago he got real angry and called me "a fat pig" and yelled, "Why can't you go on a diet?"

After several sessions in which we reviewed the week's events and her eating, Sandy started to see a relationship between Steve's comments and some of her eating:

> *Yesterday I was feeling pretty good. I had a reasonable breakfast and lunch and didn't snack all afternoon. When we ate dinner, I had the feeling that Steve was watching everything I ate. He made a few sarcastic comments about dieting and I started having urges. After dinner I told him I had to go back to the library to study, but the real reason I left was to go to Baskin-Robbins. I sat in the car and pigged out.*

Sandy's realization that her eating increased after Steve's comments helped her to see the larger pattern that characterized their relationship.

Although he didn't think of himself as obese, Steve was self-conscious about his "beer belly" and made periodic pledges to start running. A more important issue was his dissatisfaction with work. When he graduated, Steve went to work for his father so that he could save enough money to start his own business. Eight years later he was still working for his father. Each time he started looking elsewhere, his father offered him a financial incentive to stay. Although he was making a good living, Steve was unhappy and frequently complained about working for his father.

In the three months that we worked together, Sandy stopped responding to his put-downs (she called them "food fights") and gradually lost 12 pounds. Our sessions ended when she went to Hawaii.

A year later Sandy called to schedule another appointment. During their Hawaii vacation Steve intensified the food fights. Eventually Sandy gained weight. After two sessions, Sandy persuaded Steve to come in with her. Despite his misgivings, he seemed to enjoy the opportunity to talk.

I saw him individually several times and helped him explore his job, his relationship with his father, and his insecurities. Sandy was supportive and the food fights decreased. That was ten years ago. They are still married and now have two children. Although they still fight, it is rarely about eating or her weight. She comfortably maintains her weight at about 160.

The examples of Sandy and Steve and Sarah and Jerry illustrate the role that the wife's weight can play in maintaining the equilibrium in a marriage, and provide examples of unhelpful husband behaviors that are intended to restore the balance. To help you identify possible equilibrium-maintaining behaviors, I will briefly describe two basic food fight strategies and seven specific food fight techniques.

Basic Food Fight 1

According to marriage counselors Richard Stuart and Barbara Jacobson, the most effective tactic for preventing weight loss is for a husband to demand (prod, nag, or plead) that his wife lose weight. For Sandy, this was like waving a red flag in front of her. Although Steve never said it in so many words, the implication of his nagging and name calling was that Sandy was too untrustworthy or too incompetent to make her own decisions about something as simple as eating. He knew better than she did what was good for her. In addition to feeling insulted, Sandy felt unloved. Even when she started to lose weight, Steve's comments suggested that she still wasn't good enough.

Recognize that each bite you take is a personal decision you are making. Undoubtedly you know as much about the caloric value and fat content of the snack you are about to eat as your husband does. Unless you have asked for feedback, any comments he makes about your eating are intrusive. For example, if you are getting a snack from the refrigerator and your husband makes a "helpful" comment about your diet, he is putting you in a frustrating no-win situation. If you do what your husband suggests, and put the forbidden food back in the refrigerator, you are accepting that he is right and you are wrong. You feel like a child who's been caught being naughty. By putting the food back, you implicitly agree that he is a better judge of what you should eat than you are! On the other hand, if you refuse to acknowledge his superior wisdom, you are obviously weak and self-indulgent because you are eating something that isn't good for you. Either way you have just lost the food fight.

When a husband tries to control what his wife eats, he ensures that his wife will fail at any diet while he simultaneously earns points that help him "win" other marital conflicts. After overcoming Steve's defensiveness in our counseling sessions, he recognized that "reminding" Sandy about her diet (i.e., trying to control her food choices) was counterproductive. With effort, he broke this habit in several weeks. Ending Food Fight 2 took a little longer.

Basic Food Fight 2

The second basic food fight occurs when the husband makes comments which will make his wife feel bad about her body and undermine her self-esteem. A blatant example was Steve telling Sandy she looked like a "fat pig." When he wasn't so angry, Steve was much more subtle. Instead of insults, he found indirect ways of letting Sandy know that he found her body unattractive. Among the specific techniques he used were:

- Noticing and making favorable comments about other women's bodies
- Becoming an overly enthusiastic fan of thin actresses, singers, and models
- Pointing out bathing suits and revealing clothing that he wished Sandy could wear
- Finding photos of Sandy when she was thinner and telling her how much he liked the way she used to look

With Basic Food Fight 2, your husband can communicate his dissatisfaction while denying that he is pressuring you. If you try to challenge the rejection you are feeling, he will tell you, in a reasonable tone of voice, that he wasn't putting you down. He is only expressing his preferences. You can't argue with this logic because you have also said that you would like to be thinner; he's just agreeing with you. Basic Food Fight 2 leaves you frustrated, feeling unloved, and looking for something to eat.

When Steve was less dissatisfied with himself, he had less need to make Sandy feel bad. He admitted to me that, even though she wasn't thin, he still thought Sandy was very pretty. I encouraged him to let her know this.

Additional Food-Fighting Techniques

In addition to the two basic food fights, husbands can use several specific unhelpful behaviors to undermine their wife's diet. In a study of 64 married dieters, Dana Powers, a graduate student working with me, compared successful dieters who had reached their goal with less successful dieters. The less successful dieters reported that their husbands were more likely to:

1. Bring home sweets as a reward for weight loss.
2. Complain about being lonely when their wife left to exercise.
3. Insist on keeping snack foods in the house.[80]

Based on their clinical experience, Stuart and Jacobson described several additional methods that a husband can use to sabotage his wife's diet:

4. He can demand that she prepare fattening foods which are hard for her to resist.
5. He can eat snack foods in front of her and invite her to share.
6. He can go shopping and buy foods she should not eat.
7. He can complain about the cost of aerobics classes, diet foods, or health club memberships.[81]

You may remember several of these techniques from the section on chastity belts in Chapter 8. The same methods that have been used to try to ensure fidelity can be used to try to restore equilibrium.

Removing Your Weight from the Equilibrium

If you recognize any food fights from your own experience, you may be getting angry. Before you start accusing your husband, remember that an equilibrium is established over time, and both partners establish the balance without making deliberate decisions to do so. Becoming aware of the role your weight plays will allow you to remove it from the equilibrium. This can be straightforward once you understand a simple principle: *Only you can control your eating.* Unless someone ties you down and force-feeds you, or locks you up in a cell without any food, you will be the one who determines what you eat.

In Chapter 6 you set your weight reduction goal. Your decision may have included information from weight tables, and possibly feedback from others, but ultimately it is your body, your health, and your appearance so you made the decision. The same is true for each mouthful. Comments, reminders, or nagging is information from others that you *may* consider, but you will decide whether or not to eat. If someone tries to make the decision for you, you will rebel and eat just to assert your independence. You will always have the last word about your eating.

Recipes for a New Equilibrium

Since the decision is yours, you are not obligated to do what your husband wants, you are not obligated to provide an explanation to him for the decision you made, nor are you required to feel bad if you didn't do what he suggested. When this becomes clear to both you and your husband, your weight will be removed from the marital equilibrium. The six recipes presented below will help you communicate this to him.

Recipe 1

Don't let discussions get sidetracked. If you are having a disagreement about the phone bill, in-laws, or which video to rent and your weight or eating is mentioned, don't allow the focus to shift. If your husband persists, a simple response is, "That may be true, but we were talking about the phone bill. If you really want to discuss the snack I had yesterday, we can do that as soon as we are finished discussing the phone bill.''

Recipe 2

End any discussion in which your weight or eating is part of an angry outburst. If your husband calls you a name dealing with your weight, calmly end the conversation. Try not to feel hurt. It is likely he would be just as angry even if you were thin. One way of responding to an angry outburst is to say something like, ''I can see you are very angry with me. I would like to talk with you about it when you are calmer.''

Recipe 3

When your husband nags you or mentions your eating in an unhelpful way, you will have to remind him that only you can control your eating. Even if it hasn't been going well lately, you are not going to surrender each food choice to him. Instead, give a two-part response to his comments: First acknowledge his concern, and then let him know what he can do to be helpful. For example, ''You're right. I have had more urges to snack this week. Do you think you and the kids could go out for dessert, so there would be less temptation for me?''

Recipe 4

If your husband makes a favorable comment about someone else's body, or implies that he would be happier if you were thinner, don't feel bad or get defensive. Regardless of your current weight, you can also appreciate the beauty of a young actress's body. You don't have to feel bad when you remember how you looked when you were slimmer. Without any apology, agree with your husband, but add a reality check. "She does have a great body. I guess that's one reason why she got to be a famous movie star," or "I really did look good when I was in college, but we all get older."

Recipe 5

If your husband is bringing home sweets or offering you some of the high-calorie food he is eating, calmly point out the discrepancy between what he is doing now and his earlier encouragement to lose weight. For example, you could say, "The chocolate is very tempting, but I thought you wanted me to lose weight. I'm confused, which would you like? Should I eat chocolate or should I lose weight?" It may help if you can remind yourself how good it will feel to demonstrate to him that you can resist temptation. It might be more fun than eating the chocolate would be.

Recipe 6

If your husband is trying to make you feel guilty because you are spending time or money on exercise, or he misses having snack foods around the house, you will need to demonstrate that you are comfortable asking him to make these sacrifices. Don't apologize or feel guilty. Instead, acknowledge the contribution he is making and express genuine appreciation. You could say something like, "I know it's inconvenient for you when I get home late from the gym. I really appreciate the efforts you are making to help me lose weight."

If you think discussing some of these issues with your husband would be helpful, show him the "Note for Your Husband," and then make a specific request for him to change a behavior.

A Note for Your Husband

Dear Husband,

Your wife is trying to develop a new attitude toward dieting so that it will be easier for her to lose weight. One of her goals is to make sure that her weight, her dieting, and the food she eats does not get caught up in discussions of other issues. There are several simple things you can do to help:

1. Do not start discussions about her eating or weight. Even with the best intentions, she may feel like you are checking up on her. Instead, wait for her to talk about it, and then you can give her your opinions.

2. Don't let eating or weight become a part of discussions about other topics. Even if it seems related to the topic you are talking about, let her start any discussion of weight or eating.

3. Try not to make her feel bad about her weight or eating. This is not helpful. If she has done something that is annoying, let her know what she did and why you are annoyed, but don't get into a discussion about her weight.

Remember that an equilibrium established over many years will not be changed overnight. You may notice an increase in food fighting when you first try these recipes, but if you persist, you should succeed in establishing a new equilibrium which doesn't include your weight. If you have been faithfully using Recipes 1–6 and you still don't see any improvement, you might consider marriage counseling. It is possible that the issues being avoided by the focus on your weight would need professional help to be resolved.

Regardless of what you have to do to remove your weight from the marital equilibrium, you will find that it's worth the effort. You will have overcome a significant obstacle to permanent weight loss.

CHAPTER 11

The Rewarding Marriage

At this point you have developed a realistic attitude toward dieting and set reasonable weight loss goals (Chapters 5 and 6). You are working on the barriers that interfere with weight loss by detaching food from love, calming possible sexual fears, expressing annoyance without eating, and removing your weight from the marital equilibrium (Chapters 7, 8, 9, and 10). With a realistic mind-set, and without the barriers that can hold you back, it will be possible to change your eating and activity habits so that you can permanently lose weight.

Changing your eating habits doesn't require that you go "on a diet." I'm not going to give you a list of forbidden foods to avoid, or menus that you must follow. These types of interventions are always temporary. If you recall your earlier experiences, every time you went on a diet, it was followed by going off it. Instead of another repetition, let's assume that you already know, or can easily find out, which foods are high in fat and calories. What you need now is methods that will help you eat reasonable quantities of good foods (Reasons 3 and 4 in Chapter 2) without feeling deprived. The methods presented below will help you change your environment to make unhelpful eating habits less likely. We'll start with "forbidden" foods, then get into general principles for low-fat eating. Finally, you'll learn 40 specific habit-changing behaviors and a rewarding method for making them permanent.

How to Eat Chocolate

There are a few people who can simply give up a favorite food. For the rest of us, this is unrealistic. Therefore, no food is absolutely forbidden in the Recipe. If you really enjoy chocolate, ice cream, french fries, or whatever, you can have it at least occasionally, as long as you do so with the explicit purpose of enjoying it. There is no point in wasting chocolate (or any favorite food) because you are hungry and a chocolate bar is convenient. Don't eat chocolate to make yourself feel better when you are feeling bad. Don't eat chocolate because someone has set a bowl full of it on the table in front of you and it's easy to have some. Don't eat chocolate when you are doing something else that will interfere with your ability to give the chocolate the attention it deserves. Instead, when you want chocolate, plan ahead—decide when, where, and how much you would enjoy. Instead of feeling guilty, cut back on your fat consumption earlier in the day, buy a single serving of your favorite chocolate, focus on the experience, and allow yourself to enjoy it.

Eating Out

If any of your previous diets have focused on reducing your fat consumption, you know that it is not as simple as it appears. One recent study found that 88 percent of the women surveyed ate out at least once every four days. Since fast food ($149 billion per year) and vending machine food (35 billion servings per year) are higher in fat than foods you prepare at home,[82] eating out will require careful attention. The good news is that many restaurants have "healthy menus." One survey of seven chains with 4,000 restaurants in the United States found that, for most of the healthy meals, less than 30 percent of the calories came from fat.[83] Unless a hamburger with fries (1,200 calories, 58 grams of fat) is your favorite food that you have planned for, you can substitute a grilled breast of chicken (520 calories, 15 grams of fat) when you eat out.

Why You Like Fat

Despite the effects it has on your waistline, fat does have its good points. Once you understand what fat does for you, it will be easier to compensate for the fat you are going to remove from your diet.

Fat alters the texture and palatability of a food. You've probably tried some low-fat foods and found that they just don't taste as good. They may feel different in your mouth when you are eating them. People accustomed to Big Macs did not respond favorably to the McLean Burger when McDonald's introduced it several years ago. Finding low-fat substitutes that are enjoyable requires a little creativity, but it can be done. A good low-fat cookbook can help.[84]

If you have tried a low-fat diet, you may have found yourself getting hungry between meals. When you eat high-fat foods, you will stay contentedly full for a longer period than if you ate the same quantity of low-fat foods. Since low-fat foods don't "stick with you" as long, your attempts to reduce fat consumption can backfire if you're not careful.

Lucy, a 44-year-old patient, was completely baffled when she didn't lose weight after restricting her fat intake. I reviewed her self-monitoring forms and found that she ate low-fat lunches at a restaurant near her work, but prepared regular dinners for her family when she came home. Since Lucy didn't snack in the afternoon, she nibbled continuously while cooking and was still hungry when she sat down for dinner.

While fat in your diet will keep you feeling satisfied longer, it doesn't make you feel full any quicker.[85] You will eat just as much of a high-fat food before you decide that you've had enough as you would with a low-fat food. So when Lucy sat down to dinner with her family, she was hungry and ate quickly. Since it takes almost 20 minutes from the time you start eating until your brain sends the "I'm not hungry anymore" signal, her dinner more than compensated for the fat grams she avoided during lunch. I suggested that she add a low-fat afternoon snack so she wouldn't be so hungry at dinner. With the snack she had more control over her eating, ate slowly, was satisfied with smaller portions, and lost weight.

When you reduce your fat intake, there are two things to remember:

1. You will need to eat more frequently
2. You shouldn't let yourself get very hungry.

Box 22. The Most Dangerous Low-Fat Food

What food has no fat, but can be an absolute disaster? This honor goes to alcoholic beverages. Even if you avoid beer and mixed drinks, you will be consuming "empty calories" that don't provide any nutrition. According to a recent study, the calories provided by alcohol won't decrease your appetite, and may result in much more eating. According to Dr. Angelo Tremblay, the scientist who conducted the study, when you drink, "The result is higher caloric intake whether you are eating a high- or low-fat diet."[86] Alcohol can also be disinhibiting. After drinking, you may forget your usual attempts to control your eating.

Mom Was Right

One of the most common ways dieters get very hungry is by not eating breakfast. Despite your mother's admonitions to eat breakfast, you may be tempted to skip it because you're not hungry in the morning, or there isn't enough time to eat. Some dieters also skip lunch. If you skip either (or both) meals, you are going to be very hungry when you sit down to the next meal. If that meal has a heavy fat content, you will do significant damage to your diet.

Several studies have demonstrated that Mom was right about breakfast. In one study, women dieters who ate breakfast lost as much weight as dieters skipping breakfast, and were less likely to have impulsive snacks later in the day. In another study, participants who had a high-fiber cereal with milk and orange juice consumed fewer calories at lunch compared with participants eating a low-fiber breakfast. A third study showed that skipping breakfast created difficulties with problem solving and mental reasoning tasks. Participants eating a balanced breakfast (20% fat) did better than those eating an unbalanced (35% fat) breakfast.[87] These results suggest that you should eat a low-fat, high-fiber breakfast even if you are pressed for time or don't have an appetite when you wake up. Box 23 has a few suggestions that might help you eat your breakfast.

Box 23. Making Your Mother Happy

1. If you've been missing breakfast because you don't have the time, try setting the alarm 15 minutes earlier. Even if you went to bed late the night before, an extra 15 minutes' sleep will not make any difference in how tired you are, but a good breakfast will improve your mental performance, decrease your tendency to snack, and allow you to be more controlled when you eat lunch.

2. To save time, prepare your breakfast the night before.

3. If you aren't hungry when you wake up, drink a glass of fruit juice and take some food with you. When you get to work, you can eat your crackers, banana, bagel, or lightly sweetened, high-fiber cereal that you can munch right out of the box.

4. Ask your husband to have breakfast with you. Even if it isn't practical during the week, it can be a nice way to start your Saturday and Sunday.

What to Eat

Assuming you are going to eat breakfast, and not let yourself get too hungry, you can direct your attention to the fat content of the foods you eat. When you go shopping, do you check the labels to see the fat content of the foods you are buying? According to one survey, 60 percent of all shoppers are concerned with fat content.[88] While the labels provide useful information, fat awareness by itself may not produce weight loss. Some dieters interpret no-fat or low-fat on the cookie box label as permission to eat the whole box, conveniently forgetting about all the sugar inside. Even low-fat starchy foods like bread and pasta may not be so innocent. Some researchers estimate that 25 percent of the population may be insulin-resistant. For these folks, eating starches and sugar causes overproduction of insulin, which will make it more likely that these carbohydrates will be converted into body fat.[89] Most dietitians think that it is a mistake to substitute simple carbohydrates like sugar and starch for fat. Instead, diets should have larger quantities of foods like fruit, vegetables, and beans, which contain complex carbohydrates and fiber.

For most weight-conscious people, reducing fat to 30 percent or less of total calories consumed is a goal that can be met with reasonable effort. The 30 percent goal should produce weight loss, but if you are also concerned about cancer and heart disease, you will need a further reduction in fat to lower these risks.[90]

A second dietary goal should be to increase the fiber in your diet to 25–35 grams per day. This can be done by making small changes in your diet. For example, by substituting 40% bran flakes for corn flakes (an additional 4.8 grams of fiber), having a pear (4 grams of fiber) for an afternoon snack, and eating whole wheat bread rather than white bread (1.5 grams vs. 0.06 grams) you've added almost 10 grams of fiber to your diet.

How to Eat

There are many small changes in routine that, over time, will result in weight loss. When these changes become habits, there will be fewer food cues in your environment to tempt you. Your new habits will decrease the speed of eating so you will consume less without feeling deprived. Although it takes a little practice to change an old habit, after several weeks the new habit becomes automatic and the reduction in your eating can be permanent.

Most of the techniques on the following list were developed for behavioral weight control programs,[91] although a few have been suggested by colleagues and former patients. Several may look familiar to you because they appeared earlier in one of the boxes. If you aren't already using the technique, now would be a good time to start. Read through the list, review your self-monitoring cards (if you haven't been faithfully self-monitoring, reread Chapter 6, and then start now), and decide which of the techniques are most important for you.

In the space provided, rate each technique. If it is totally irrelevant to your circumstances, for example, the technique deals with cooking and you don't cook, give it a 0. If you are already using a technique regularly, give it a 1 and give yourself a pat on the back! If the technique applies to a situation that you encounter, and you usually don't do what is suggested, give it a 2. If it applies to a situation that frequently occurs, but you're not sure if you use the technique, or you think it would be too difficult or impractical to use, give it a 2 anyway. The reward system you will be using will help to increase your motivation so that it will be less difficult or impractical. Here's the list:

Eating Avoidance

_____ 1. Never make phone calls from the kitchen.

_____ 2. For routine trips like going shopping or to work, find a route that does not pass bakeries, ice cream stores, fast-food restaurants, or the cookie shop in the mall.

_____ 3. Do boring chores in food-free environments.

_____ 4. In situations where you would be tempted

to eat (watching TV, for example), chew gum and do something with your hands.

Shopping and Meal Planning

_____ 1. Prepare a shopping list of low-fat foods, and buy foods only from the list. If this is difficult, bring only enough money for the foods on the list.

_____ 2. Never shop on an empty stomach.

_____ 3. When shopping, avoid the aisles and checkout lanes with displays of candy and desserts.

_____ 4. Don't go shopping with young children who will demand snacks and candy that they see on the shelves.

_____ 5. Let other family members buy their own snacks and desserts. Have them put their name on the snacks so that you are not tempted to sample them.

_____ 6. If you must buy snacks for other family members, buy snacks that they like but you don't.

_____ 7. If your husband or children strongly object to low-fat meals, save most of your fat grams for meals you eat with them. Plan very low-fat meals when you eat by yourself.

_____ 8. If you are going to have a high-fat treat—ice cream, for example—plan for it and eat it out of the house. You will be less likely to buy more than one serving if you eat in public and don't bring it into the house.

_____ 9. If you must have snacks in the house, buy them in single-serving packages.

Food Storage

_____ 1. Keep all the food in the kitchen (no snacks in the living room, treats in your dresser drawer, or munchies in the glove compartment in the car).

_____ 2. Store high-fat foods in opaque containers and keep them in the back of the refrigerator, freezer, or pantry.

_____ 3. Make low-fat snacks easy to get (e.g., keep applesauce or small, washed carrots in clear wrap toward the front of the refrigerator).

Food Preparation and Serving

_____ 1. Make sure that any tasting or sampling gets recorded on your self-monitoring forms.

_____ 2. Chew gum while you cook.

_____ 3. Ask other family members to help with food preparation or take turns cooking.

_____ 4. If you cook in large quantities, put the excess in containers and freeze for a future meal before you start to serve today's meal.

_____ 5. Serve the food directly onto plates in the kitchen. Don't put serving bowls or platters on the table where you'll be eating. If you really want a second helping, get up from the table and go into the kitchen to get it.

Eating

_____ 1. Do all your at-home eating, including snacks, sitting at one place at the kitchen or dining room table. Never eat standing up.

_____ 2. Make eating a singular activity. Turn off the television, don't read, and don't talk on the phone while eating.

_____ 3. Drink at least two large glasses of water before each meal.

_____ 4. Try eating with your nondominant hand.

_____ 5. Put your knife and fork down after each bite and don't pick them up again until after you have swallowed.

_____ 6. Pause in the middle of the meal and put your knife and fork down. With half of your food still in front of you, continue conversing but don't eat for one minute.

_____ 7. At least once during the meal, direct your attention to the experience of eating. Notice the taste (sweet? bitter? spicy?), the texture, and the temperature of the food you are eating. Try to identify the seasonings.

_____ 8. Do not clean your plate. Leave a little food on the plate.

_____ 9. When you are finished eating, excuse yourself (although if you have been eating slowly, you won't be the first to finish) and get up from the table.

_____ 10. Brush and floss your teeth immediately after eating to reduce the chances of additional eating.

Cleaning Up

_____ 1. Have your husband and children clean the table and put their own dishes into the dishwasher or sink.

_____ 2. Have your husband or children put the

leftovers in opaque containers, and when possible, put the containers in the freezer.

Eating Out

_____ 1. Plan ahead. Choose a restaurant that offers low-fat items on the menu.

_____ 2. Consider sharing the entrée and ordering an extra salad.

_____ 3. Ask the waiter for a "doggie bag." Before you start to eat, divide the food into the portion you'll eat and the portion you'll take home.

Parties and Social Events

_____ 1. At cocktail parties and buffets, stand on the other side of the room with your back to the food table.

_____ 2. If your husband is participating, ask for his help planning your eating. For example, at a buffet you could have him serve you.

_____ 3. At informal parties, bring your own low-fat snacks.

_____ 4. If you feel like you need to have something in your hand, carry a glass of diet soda or water with ice cubes.

Now go through the list of techniques that you rated 2, and circle at least three, but no more than five, that you will work on first. If you would like, get your husband's input, but you make the final decision. After two weeks, you will review your progress and add additional techniques from the list.

If your husband is participating, ask him to read the "Note for Your Husband," which explains how he can help. Since changing behavior is easier when the new behavior is rewarded, it will be important to develop rewards that you can use and a contract that will specify how and when you will be rewarded. Box 24 presents a list of suggestions, and some spaces for you to write additional ideas. Be creative in planning rewards; just be sure you don't get too grandiose. Although a Fifth Avenue or Rodeo Drive shopping spree would be nice, the rewards should be simple pleasures that are not too expensive or time-consuming. Many of the rewards on the list are nice things your husband can do for you or that you can do together. After he has read the "Note for Your Husband," you can ask him to help add to the list.

If your husband isn't participating, it might not be as much fun, but you can still reward yourself with some of the items on the list. For example, it is still enjoyable to have flowers or a magazine about one of your hobbies even if you buy them for yourself.

Box 24. Rewards for Behavior Change

1. Buy flowers or pick flowers from the yard.
2. Send a greeting card.
3. Give or receive a massage or backrub.
4. Go to the movies, a play, a concert, or a sporting event together.
5. Have your spouse do one of your routine chores.
6. Make a phone call just to see how your spouse's day is going.
7. Play cards or a favorite game.
8. Buy a magazine about one of your interests or hobbies.
9. Go with your spouse to a meeting or event dealing with one of your interests.
10. Go dancing.
11. Find a lover's lane and park.

12. Go to church or synagogue together.

13. Take a shower or bath together.

14. Go to a lecture, or take an adult education class or workshop together.

15. Go window shopping.

16. Send a fax or e-mail to your spouse at work.

17. Buy reasonably priced makeup or fashion accessory.

18. _____

19. _____

20. _____

A Note for Your Husband

Dear Husband,

Your wife is going to be changing some of her eating habits. You can help by being supportive and participating, when appropriate, in the new behaviors that will be required. She will show you a list of behavior changes and ask your help in working on several. After discussing these changes, you can help by:

1. Set a good example by modeling the desired behavior. For example, if she is trying to eat slowly, you can eat slowly too. Try to avoid eating in front of her other than at mealtimes.

2. Focus on behavior change rather than weight loss. Weight loss may not immediately follow behavior change even if she has been working hard at it. When your wife has been making progress with behavior

change, compliment her even if there hasn't been any weight loss.

3.   When you think she may be tempted to snack, try to engage her in some activity that is incompatible with eating. Show her something you've been working on, discuss an article you've read, or go for a walk so that she is distracted until the urge to eat passes.

4.   Reward a desirable behavior change. In addition to praising her (see No. 2 above), you can arrange small rewards. Box 24 in this chapter presents a list of inexpensive or free pleasurable activities that can be used as rewards, and Box 25 is a contract that specifies her immediate goals and the rewards she will get when she has accomplished these goals. Using rewards and the contract will increase her motivation to change her eating habits.

Have you been concerned about your own weight, or is there another behavior you want to change (maybe watch less television or spend more time with your children)? Both you and your wife can use the contract to reward each other for desirable behavior changes. If there aren't any behaviors you want to work on right now, then the contract can focus exclusively on your wife's goals; the choice is yours. In either case, you can use the contract presented in Box 25 to define what you both will do to reward the desired behavior changes.

A Contract

Box 25 presents a contract that you can use to specify the changes you will be making and the rewards that you will receive. Don't get turned off by the word "contract." This is not a legal document so you don't need to worry about each word. What the contract will do is to make your good intentions tangible and increase your motivation to follow through.

If your husband is participating, ask for his input in choosing at least three goals and two rewards. Don't be limited by the lists in this chapter. If you have an eating habit that you would like to change, or a specific temptation that you would like to resist, include it in the contract. Your husband can use the contract to change one or more of his behaviors, if he is motivated to change. If not, he can still help you with your eating habits. Just leave the spaces for his behavior blank.

If your husband is not participating, you can still use the contract to specify which behaviors you are going to work on, and how you will reward yourself. After you have filled in your behavior changes and rewards, sign and date it on the bottom. Then tell a trusted friend what your behavior change goals are and how you plan to reward yourself when they have been accomplished. Although the friend doesn't need to sign the contract, by telling another person about it, you will make it more likely that you will follow through.

Box 25. Behavioral Contract

This contract between _____ (husband) and _____ (wife) specifies what each will do to help the other make desired changes in behavior. Starting today, and continuing until _____, the wife will make the following changes in her eating behaviors:

1. _____

2. _____

3. _____

4. _____

5. _____

If, at the end of the day week (circle one), she presents evidence that she has made the changes listed above, she will be rewarded by:

1. _____

2. _____

If the husband is trying to change his behavior, he will make the following specific change(s):

1. _____

2. _____

3. _____

If, at the end of the day week (circle one), he presents evidence that he has made the changes listed above, the wife will reward him by:

1. _____

2. _____

```
_____        _____
Wife                         Husband


_____
Date
```

Continue with the contract for two weeks and then evaluate which of the new behaviors have become easier, and which still need work. Write up a new contract adding behaviors from the list while keeping those that need more work. If you have done well, you can increase the number of behaviors you will work on in your second contract. If you find that the rewards you've chosen are losing their effectiveness, pick new ones. If your husband is using the contract to change his behaviors, he can make similar modifications.

Jeff and Margaret

Remember Jeff and Margaret, the couple described in Chapter 4? She was a 36-year-old accountant, he was a 44-year-old contractor, and both were overweight. When Margaret started, Jeff was working out of town during the week so his participation was minimal. Once he returned, Jeff became more curious about what Margaret was doing. He agreed to help her with her contract, but wasn't interested in changing any of his behaviors. Margaret's first contract included several of the techniques intended to decrease the speed of her eating. At a session several months later, Jeff explained:

Margaret was putting her knife and fork down, and taking a break in the middle of the meal. I felt foolish rushing through dinner and being the first one finished. Before I knew it, I was eating slowly too, and it wasn't hard to do. Then I figured, I could stand to lose some weight, so we had a talk and wrote a new contract which included some changes that I needed to make. Aside from the weight that we've both lost, the best part is that we figured out a couple of ways of rewarding each other that weren't on your list.

Jeff grinned but did not elaborate any further. It was clear that he was quite happy with their weight losses, and the improvement in their relationship.

CHAPTER 12

Doing It Together

In any workshop on weight, when I mention the word "exercise," several of the participants will squirm uncomfortably, laugh nervously, or groan. Especially if they have been struggling with their weight since childhood, the idea of strenuous physical activity produces visible discomfort. How about you? Are you starting to feel uncomfortable knowing what this chapter is about? Are you expecting a sermon intending to shame you into exercising? You can relax. Although this chapter is about physical activity, you don't need to feel uneasy. You won't have to sweat (unless you want to) or feel guilty for not sweating. Instead you will understand why you have bad feelings about exercise and what you can do that will make you feel good.

Why Bother?

Chapter 2 presented evidence that physical inactivity is one of the most common reasons for weight gain. You will recall that becoming active promotes weight loss three ways: using energy to do the activity, increasing metabolic rate for some time after you've finished the activity, and increasing your muscle tissue, which uses more energy (calories). Whenever I describe these findings, someone will object, "That may be true, but if I started to exercise, I would just become hungrier and eat more." For most overweight women this is not likely. The results of several studies suggest that if you increase your physical activity to a low or moderate intensity, your appetite will decrease rather than increase. You have to exercise vigorously before your appetite increases.[92]

Low- to moderate-intensity exercise has health and psychological benefits independent of weight loss. Regular exercise, even if it is not strenuous, reduces your risk of coronary heart disease, osteoporosis, and some types of cancer.[93] One study of 13,000 men and women followed over eight years found that, in contrast to subjects who were very unfit, subjects who participated in low levels of physical activity had very significant reductions in health risks.[94] It's been estimated that as many as 250,000 deaths each year result from a lack of regular physical activity.[95] Even if you weren't trying to lose weight, 30 minutes of daily activity would be worthwhile just for the health benefits. The same is true for your husband, regardless of his weight.

The psychological benefits of exercise are more immediate. Many studies have shown reductions in depression and improvements in mood and self-esteem resulting from exercise.[96] Frequently I can see the difference in my patients after following an exercise routine for a few weeks. Many seem more enthusiastic and energetic. Dr. Kelly

Brownell, a prominent obesity researcher, thinks that an active lifestyle makes weight control easier because of the improvements in self-esteem, body image, and the ability to deal with negative moods.[97]

Several studies show that people who exercise are more likely to maintain their weight losses. One study compared overweight women who lost weight and maintained the loss with women who lost but then regained weight. Ninety percent of the maintainers, but only 34 percent of the regainers, exercised regularly.[98] If you are going to put the effort into losing weight, you will need to exercise to maintain the loss.

Why bother to exercise? These findings have clear implications for you:

- Physical activity will decrease, not increase, your appetite.
- Physical activity reduces your health risks.
- Physical activity will improve your mood and self-esteem.
- Physical activity will help you lose weight.
- Physical activity is necessary for you to maintain weight loss.

A Personal Note

Although I was somewhat overweight as a child, I rode my bicycle and played ball with the kids in the neighborhood. By the time I got to high school I was avoiding gym whenever possible and rarely played sports. In college and early adulthood I became a typical couch potato. It's only a slight exaggeration to say that my longest walks were from the living room to the refrigerator. After several years of telling myself I didn't have the time, and it would be too boring anyway, I joined a fitness club. That was 16 years ago and I'm still at it. I can't tell you that I've always enjoyed the experience. During the first year, I remember my son asking which was my favorite exercise. I answered, "Pushing the door on the way out."

At the age of 54, I still lift weights and use a stair-stepper at the gym, and walk 20 minutes to work. I don't always look forward to working out, but knowing how much better I will feel when I'm finished is enough to keep me coming back, even when I have a plausible excuse for skipping my workout. In addition to keeping my weight under control, I have less back and knee pain, and have more energy after exercising.

Why It's So Hard to Exercise

In Chapter 2 you compared your current physical activities and daily routines with your activity level as a teen or young adult. If, like most dieters, you found a big difference, what happened? If there are so many benefits, why is it so hard to exercise? Several factors, ranging from broad social changes to deeply personal psychological issues, are responsible.

When you were younger, you got up from the sofa to change the channel, wound the car windows up by hand, got out of the car to open the garage door, and so on. Even typing with a manual typewriter used more energy than word processing with a computer. All the technological advances of the past few years have allowed you to conserve energy. In addition to the advent of numerous labor-saving devices, your daily routine changed as you got married and settled into adulthood. If you give it a little thought, you will be able to remember physical activities you no longer do. What may be less obvious than the changes in your routine, and all the labor-saving devices you use, are the subtle psychological processes that make it less likely that you will be active.

Are You Lazy?

Is laziness the real reason you don't exercise? Many overweight women (and their husbands) attribute their inactivity to laziness, and then feel guilty about being lazy. This unhelpful overgeneralization makes it less likely that you will understand, and resolve, the concerns that prevent you from becoming more active.

Chrissy, a 27-year-old, part-time student is a good example. She was tall, weighed 185 pounds, and was a self-described "couch potato." Adam, her live-in boyfriend, played golf, worked out at a fitness center, and was trying to get Chrissy to join a coed softball team with him. She seemed embarrassed as she told me about her reluctance, especially since she thought playing ball might help her to lose weight.

CHRISSY: I played sports until my junior year in high school, but now I won't do anything athletic because I'm fat. I sweat a lot and it feels gross, so I don't do any exercise. I know I should, but I don't because I'm too lazy.

DR. A: How do you know you're lazy?

CHRISSY: Well, I'm lazy because I don't exercise.

DR. A: Let's see, you don't exercise because you're "too lazy," and you know you're lazy because you don't exercise. That sounds like circular reasoning to me, but you also said you "sweat a lot and it feels gross." Can you explain?

CHRISSY: I went with Adam to the gym where he works out a couple of times. I tried the treadmill and

	the exercise bicycle. I was sweaty and out of breath after a few minutes. I couldn't finish.
DR. A:	Other than being sweaty and out of breath, were there any problems?
CHRISSY:	Yeah, I felt foolish.
DR. A:	Tell me about that.
CRISSY:	Well, you know I don't exactly look like a cheerleader. There were all these cute college girls with perfect bodies, and I'm wearing a sweat suit to try to cover my stomach and my butt. I thought everyone was looking at me. I felt awkward and out of place.
DR. A:	So when you exercise, you feel self-conscious, sweaty, and out of breath. It seems that what you call lazy is really just a fear of being uncomfortable and embarrassed. If we could figure out a way to exercise without being uncomfortable, would you be interested?

Although she was a little skeptical, Chrissy was very interested. After we worked out an exercise program that she could follow comfortably, she stopped thinking about herself as lazy.

Avoiding Unpleasantness

Almost everyone who has been struggling with their weight has had repeated bad experiences with physical activity. How many of the following have you experienced?

- Ridicule or feeling embarrassed after you did poorly in a competitive sport—for example, striking out while playing softball or being the last one chosen for the team.
- Feeling self-conscious about your body because the

clothing you had to wear (leotard, shorts, or swim-suit) drew attention to your body.
- Feeling clumsy and uncoordinated, or not being able to keep up with your peers.
- Feeling nervous because you were the center of attention; everyone was looking at you.
- Sweating profusely, gasping for breath, or feeling body aches and pains.
- Discouragement after vigorous exercise didn't produce any weight loss, or exercise directed to a specific part of the body did not decrease its size.

If you have had any of these experiences, why would you want to exercise? After all, how many people do you know who choose to put themselves in situations where they will be physically uncomfortable and feel humiliated? Instead of viewing your reluctance to exercise as a sign of laziness, it is more reasonable to see it as an attempt to avoid unpleasantness.

The good news is that you are not in high school anymore. You don't have to deal with gym classes, locker rooms, skimpy outfits, and gym teachers egging you on while other kids are watching. Now you can increase your physical activity by a combination of small habit changes that become automatic, and painless exercise sessions that become part of your daily routine. You can avoid the unpleasant experiences of the past by choosing an exercise routine that is not competitive, doesn't require that you wear revealing clothing, doesn't depend on your coordination or physical strength, doesn't focus everyone's attention on you, and doesn't require that you overexert yourself. You can avoid disappointing weigh-ins when you understand how activity affects your weight. You will pick a routine that you can do comfortably; the only problem is finding the time.

No Time, Too Tired for Exercise

Maybe you don't think you're lazy—you'd really like to exercise, but it's just that you don't have enough time. Not having the time is the most common rationalization for not exercising. With the possible exception of prisoners held in solitary confinement, the rest of us make choices about how we spend our time. Even with demanding jobs, we are still making these choices. To put your decisions about time for exercise in perspective, it might help to remember that both Bill Clinton and George Bush run despite the demands of their job. More common folk find ways of integrating activity into their daily routines so that they still take care of business. They walk on their lunch hour, put their toddlers on seats when they ride their bikes, or use the child care where they do their aerobics class. For most people, the easiest way of finding time to exercise is to turn off the television. One study found that more television viewing was associated with less physical activity and more snacking,[99] so decreasing time spent watching television can have several benefits.

Even if you have the time, when you're tired, the thought of exercise can be overwhelming. Usually the weariness you feel at the end of the day is more mental than physical. You will find that, after you push yourself to start, you're no longer tired. If you're a little skeptical, try a little activity the next time you're feeling fatigued. See if you don't have more energy when you've finished than you had before starting.

Exercising or not exercising is a choice that we all make. To help you choose, let's divide your activity into two parts: the things you can do to increase physical movement while you do your usual activities, and time devoted specifically to exercise. If you can find an exercise routine that doesn't cause discomfort or embarrassment, and add motivation from rewards you or your husband will provide, it will be easy to choose to be more active. Let's start with your daily routine.

Daily Routines

Making small changes in your routines won't produce noticeable weight losses, so if you run to the scale to check your progress, you're going to be disappointed. Instead, remind yourself that the benefits will be gradual weight loss, prevention of further weight gain, and improvements in mood and health.

About ten years ago, I was having a casual conversation with Mark, a recently hired professor at the university. He was complaining about the hassles he had trying to park on campus. He bought a parking decal at the beginning of the semester, but usually all the spots in the parking lot near his building were taken. He would then drive around the lot waiting for someone to leave, becoming increasingly stressed as the time for his class approached. If he couldn't find a spot, he would park illegally, hope that he didn't get a ticket, and go to class. The next semester he decided to park on a residential street five blocks from his office. The walk took him about seven minutes each way. This didn't take any longer than trying to park in the lot, and the walk left him feeling less stressed (even when it was raining).

I was talking to Mark recently and reminded him of our conversation ten years ago. We calculated the consequences of the change in his parking routine. At the time he weighed about 180 pounds, so 15 minutes of brisk walking each day used approximately 108 calories. Theoretically, Mark's brisk walks could have produced a reduction of about 5.5 pounds a year, if everything else was unchanged. Since Mark currently weighs between 175–177, we figured that his walking helped to prevent the weight gain that usually comes with getting older. Although it's hard to quantify improvements in mood, Mark said he now enjoys the walks. He sees them as a nice interlude that helps him to make the transition from home to work, and work to home.

Think about your routine. Where can you add some physical movement? It can be small changes: Stand instead of sit, or walk instead of stand. Even small body movements like fidgeting can help.[100] According to one calculation, fidgeting may use as much as 800 calories per day! Being nervous by itself doesn't consume calories—it is the body movements you make—so you can fidget even when you're feeling relaxed. Just don't expect to see results if you step on the scale at the end of the day. Whether you choose to fidget or not, the goal is to use every opportunity to move your body. Box 26 presents a few suggestions for increasing physical movement.

Box 26. Adding Movement to Your Day

Use a portable phone and walk while you talk.

Don't pile up items at the foot of the stairs, make several trips.

Use stairs rather than an elevator or escalator.

Get off the bus one stop earlier and walk.

Dance to music while doing housework.

Hang laundry outside instead of using a dryer.

Do some of your desk work standing up.

Pace while conversing or teaching a class.

Walk your children to school.

Ride a bicycle when doing errands.

Rake leaves instead of using a blower.

Don't phone coworkers, walk to their office.

Iron while watching television.

Park on far side of the parking lot.

Wash your car by hand.

Play active games with children.

Work in the yard or garden.

Use a bathroom on a different floor.

Walk the dog more often.

Don't use the television remote.

Have sex more frequently.

Vacuum more often.

Mix dough by hand.

Cut wood for the fireplace.

Do a few jumping jacks.

Now think about your routines at home and work. Can you think of any labor-saving patterns that you can change? What else can you do to increase your movement every day? Write in at least four changes you will make to increase activity in your daily routines.

1. _____   4. _____

2. _____   5. _____

3. _____   6. _____

No Pain, Big Gain

In addition to the changes you will make in your daily routine, you should plan one or more moderate activities with the goal of doing 30 minutes of activity every day. You can do the 30 minutes once a day, or divide it into several shorter periods—whichever is more convenient for you. To help plan an exercise routine, go back to the section "Avoiding Unpleasantness" and identify which of the bad experiences with exercise you have had. For example, if you feel self-conscious wearing revealing clothing, there is no point in signing up for an aerobics class that requires you to wear leotards. While it would still be helpful to improve your body image (see Box 17 in Chapter 8), to get started, pick an exercise that you can do comfortably now.

To help pick an activity, get to know yourself. Base your plans on *your* likes and dislikes rather than an arbitrary idea of what you should do. Can you see yourself doing the activity for a year, or more? There is no point in planning exercise that is too vigorous and that will be abandoned after several frustrating attempts. Instead start with an activity, intensity, and duration that you can manage comfortably, and then you can gradually increase the intensity or duration.

Keep in mind that you will be disappointed if you pick an exercise with the goal of changing a specific part of your body. For example, sit-ups will strengthen your abdominal muscles, but will not make you lose the fat around your middle. As you become more active and improve your eating habits, you'll see a reduction in your waistline, even if you never do a sit-up.

Consider where you will do your exercise. While many active people enjoy health or fitness clubs, one study found that sedentary women participating in a weight control program which included a home-based walking routine persisted longer, and lost more weight than women who did their walking on a treadmill in a clinic.[101]

The Surgeon General's Report on Physical Activity and Health presented guidelines for moderate activity that can significantly improve health.[102] Box 27 lists a few moderate-intensity activities with the time that would be required to meet the Surgeon General's recommendations for physical activity. Most of these activities don't draw attention to your body or require any athletic skill or physical strength.

Box 27. Surgeon General's Recommendations

Activity	Minutes
Swimming laps (low–moderate effort)	17
Jogging	19
Bicycling (less than 10 mph)	22
Chopping wood	22
Mowing lawn	24
Aerobic dancing (low-impact)	26
Brisk walking (4.5 mph)	29
Gardening	33
Horseback riding	33
Normal walking (3 mph)	38
Food shopping with a cart	38
Volleyball (noncompetitive)	44
Carpet or floor sweeping	53
Washing dishes standing	57

If you are feeling overwhelmed by the length of time recommended, remember that this is a goal that you can work toward. Start at a level that you can do comfortably, even if it's only a five-minute walk around the block, and do it every day. Every few minutes take the "talk test." You should be able to carry on a conversation while you are exercising. If you can't, slow down until you can. Once your routine has been established, you will find, almost automatically, you will want to do it a little longer or a little faster, or both. Eventually you will reach your time and intensity goals if you get into the exercise habit, but you won't get into the habit if you try to push yourself too hard in the beginning.

The Walk

For most of my patients, walking is the mainstay of their exercise plan. Other than a pair of comfortable shoes, it doesn't require special equipment or clothing. It can be done anytime, almost anywhere. It is noncompetitive, doesn't require strength or coordination, doesn't draw attention to your body, it can be done without sweating or breathing hard (although some people enjoy working up a sweat). Once you get in the habit, you will find that a walk enriches your day. For example, Mark used his walks to make the transition between home and work so he felt prepared when he arrived. Other benefits that patients have described include: an opportunity to plan the day's activities, an opportunity to daydream creatively, a relief from stress and tension, being outdoors enjoying nature, a few minutes of solitude and privacy, an opportunity to meet neighbors, a chance to have an uninterrupted conversation with a friend, and an opportunity to experience one's body in a positive way. It's not essential that you walk every day. When you plan your exercise for the week, feel free to mix and match. For example, you could do your weekly food shopping on Tuesday, go bicycle riding with your kids on Saturday, and take a brisk walk on the other days. Just be sure that you plan your weekly exercise schedule in advance. You shouldn't have to make daily decisions. You will know, if today is Wednesday, you're going for a walk at 8:30 A.M.

Getting Motivated

Although some people like the peace of a solitary walk or enjoy listening to music on their Walkman, others use their walks as an opportunity to socialize. Even if you are walking briskly, you still should be able to carry on a conversation, so you can invite a friend, a coworker, or your husband to walk with you. At work, if you regularly meet with a coworker, ask if she would like to walk while having your meeting. If you don't know anyone who would be interested in walking with you, put up a notice looking for a lunch time walking partner or mention your interest at the PTA meeting, church groups, or neighborhood organizations. You might make some new friends in the process and forget that you are getting exercise while you are socializing.

The likeliest candidate for a walking partner is your husband. If your husband is participating, show him the letter following and then complete the activity contract. If he doesn't participate in physical activity with you, you can still use the contract and the incentives you identified in Chapter 11 to be rewarded for your increased activity.

A Note for Your Husband

Dear Husband,

Research demonstrates that increasing physical activity is the single most important change a person can make to lose weight, and is almost essential to maintain weight losses once they have been accomplished. Although exercise does not produce immediate weight loss, even small increases in physical activity will gradually help, in addition to reducing other health risks and improving your wife's psychological well-being. You can read earlier sections of this chapter if you would like a more complete discussion of these findings.

If your wife has been physically inactive for some time, it may be difficult for her to get into the habit of daily activity. This is where you can help. If you have also been inactive, you will benefit from participating with her regardless of your weight, since your health risks and well-being will also improve with daily exercise. On the other hand, if you are currently active, either at work or with sports or hobbies, you can help her without disrupting your own activities. Keep in mind that she will be more likely to persist, if she tries moderate-intensity activities, rather than vigorous exercises which require extreme effort and sweat. Read the list of activities to see which would be fun if the two of you did them together. Discuss with your wife:

1. The activities you will do together
2. The days and times you will do them
3. The necessary arrangements (child care, for example) that need to be made

Then complete the contract in Box 28.

If you are not going to exercise with her, you can still help by rewarding her when she does her exercising. You can use the contract in Box 28; just leave the section for husband's physical activity blank.

Box 28. Behavioral Contract

This contract between _____ (husband) and _____ (wife) specifies what each will do to help the other make desired changes in behavior. Starting today, and continuing until _____, the wife will make the following changes in her physical activity:

1. Every Sunday she will___ from _____ to _____.

2. Every Monday she will___ from _____ to _____.

3. Every Tuesday she will___ from _____ to _____.

4. Every Wednesday she will___ from _____ to _____.

5. Every Thursday she will___ from _____ to _____.

6. Every Friday she will___ from _____ to _____.

7. Every Saturday she will___ from _____ to _____.

If the husband is participating in some physical activities with the wife:

1. Every Sunday he will___ from _____ to _____.

2. Every Monday he will____ from _____ to _____.

3. Every Tuesday he will____ from _____ to _____.

4. Every Wednesday he will_ from _____ to _____.

5. Every Thursday he will____ from _____ to _____.

6. Every Friday he will_____ from _____ to _____.

7. Every Saturday he will____ from _____ to _____.

If the husband is not going to participate in physical activities with his wife, and she has made the changes listed above, she will be rewarded by:

1. _____

2. _____

_____   _____
Wife   Husband

_____
Date

Chrissy's Exercise Program

Chrissy, the self-described couch potato, decided that maybe she wasn't so lazy after all, and would try to develop an exercise routine. Since Adam had been wanting Chrissy to exercise, he was a willing—in fact, overenthusiastic—

partner. Before Chrissy had finished telling him about our discussion, Adam was going to sign her up for softball and was planning her exercise routine at his fitness club. Firmly, she told Adam that there was no point in starting a routine that she wouldn't be able to maintain, so he would have to play softball and work out without her. She was going to start by adding activity to her routine, and taking a daily walk. She asked if he'd like to walk with her and help her with a contract. After some discussion they agreed on a contract that stipulated that she would:

1.   Hang the clothes out to dry when it wasn't raining (Adam readily agreed since this would save on electricity bills).

2.   Ride her bicycle to class.

3.   Walk up stairs to all classes on the second or third floor.

4.   Play music and dance while doing housework.

5.   Walk for a minimum of 10 minutes in the morning.

Adam agreed to:

1.   Walk with her on days when he was home in the morning.

2.   Give her a back rub when she hung the clothes to dry, or rode her bicycle to class.

Chrissy and Adam did not follow the contract perfectly. Several times, when it was raining, Chrissy didn't ride her bicycle to class, and in the beginning she missed some of her morning walks. Adam tried not to criticize, and helped rewrite the contract so that she didn't have to ride the bike on rainy days and could choose one day each week to skip her walk. Having Adam's support and being able to rewrite the contract helped Chrissy avoid feeling trapped, and enabled her to continue when she was tempted to give up. Within three months the walks and bike riding had become habits. She felt good about her exercise, stopped thinking of herself as lazy, and lost weight.

CHAPTER 13

Deadly Detours

Stephanie called to tell me she wasn't coming to the group meeting tomorrow. When I asked her why, she became flustered and started to make up an excuse. I interrupted her and asked:

DR. A: You sound upset. Are you sure there isn't
              something else going on?
STEPHANIE: I don't know, nothing seems to be working.
DR. A: Tell me what happened.
STEPHANIE: Well, I thought I was doing so well. I had
              lost fifteen pounds, and was walking every
              day, but last week I was home sick for four
              days, so I couldn't go for my walk. On
              Wednesday I went out with my friends at
              work and they were all having dessert. I
              got teased about my diet, so I just gave in
              and had a big piece of pie. Then I got
              discouraged. I didn't pay attention to what

I was eating yesterday. I've really blown it.
I was just fooling myself when I thought
that, this time, I really was going to lose
weight.

Stephanie has hit two detours, and has had a lapse.
What happens next will determine her success or failure
at weight loss. Before I tell you what happened to Stephanie, let's look at the inevitable setbacks that dieters
encounter.

Detours on the Road to Permanent Weight Loss

One goal of the Recipe is to change your thinking about
dieting. Instead of the yo-yo pattern of dieting, you know
that weight loss is an ongoing process with new behaviors
that help control eating and increase activity. With practice, the new behaviors become habits that are part of your
daily routine. Things are going well and your weight is
decreasing until something in your world changes. You
are now at an intersection. The new circumstances are a
potential detour that can lead you away from your weight
loss lifestyle, or if you have a Relapse Prevention Plan
in place, you can avoid the detour and continue making
progress.

In this chapter we will examine the most common
changes that can easily lead you to take a detour. You will
then develop a plan that you can implement when you see
the first signs of a detour. If you are going to put the effort
into changing your eating and exercise habits, you will
need to protect your investment by planning ahead so that
you can avoid the detours that result in regained weight.
Although almost any change in routine can be a potential
detour, some of the most common are listed here.

Detour 1: The Holiday Season

Probably the most predictable situation that can produce a detour is the holiday season. From the end of November through the beginning of the new year, there are many opportunities to abandon your new eating habits and give up your exercise routine.

In most families, Thanksgiving dinner requires overeating. If you try to adhere to your new eating habits, you will feel out of place. To fully participate, you need to have seconds of everything, but Thanksgiving is only the opening of the eating season. Next comes a series of holiday parties at work and with friends, followed by dinners on Christmas Eve and Christmas Day, culminating in New Year's Eve parties and New Year's Day get-togethers.

One study of dieters in a weight loss program clearly demonstrated the effects of the holidays. The researchers compared weight gains during holiday weeks vs. nonholiday weeks. The dieters gained five times as much during the holiday weeks.[103] Although birthdays, weddings, and family gatherings don't last as long as the holiday season, these celebrations also involve food and may present similar dangers.

Exercise routines are also difficult to maintain during the holiday season. Even if party going does not interfere with your routine, the weather might. Nature conspires to keep you indoors; it gets colder, wetter, and darker earlier.

Avoiding the holiday season detour is difficult, so don't get discouraged if you are having problems. It may be that you will be doing well if you maintain your weight in November and December, and resume your weight loss in January. Even if you don't expect to lose, you should not feel that you can completely abandon your weight control efforts. The best way of preparing yourself for the holidays is to get into the self-monitoring habit well before Thanksgiving. A recent study demonstrated that dieters who are consistent in their self-monitoring throughout the year do better during the holidays. The consistent self-monitors continued monitoring through the holidays and did not gain weight, while inconsistent self-monitors did less monitoring during the holidays and gained weight.[104]

Detour 2: Social Pressure

Chapter 10 described many of the tactics husbands can use to interfere with their wife's weight loss. Unfortunately, husbands aren't the only people who can disrupt your progress. When your weight loss becomes noticeable, you may start to hear discouraging comments from friends, siblings, or parents who are jealous or feel threatened by your success. At lunch, a friend may encourage you to have dessert, your mother may express concern that your weight loss is unhealthy, or you may get teased about your rigid adherence to your exercise routine. Sometimes, without meaning any harm, a group of friends, might encourage you to join in when they are eating high-fat foods. For example, Stephanie found it hard to resist the social pressure when her friends were ordering desserts. She didn't want to be the spoilsport who wasn't participating.

Detour 3: Vacations

Going on vacation presents twin dangers. The first is that many vacations feature eating as a major part of the experience. It's hard to maintain your low-fat diet when you take a cruise or go to an all-inclusive resort that presents you with huge buffets three times a day, along with several lavish snacks. If you decide to go sightseeing instead, you'll be doing all of your eating in restaurants where you'll be tempted to overindulge in the local specialties.

The second danger is that a vacation, even if it only lasts for one week, disrupts your patterns. After a week when you are not keeping your routines, it will be easy to come home and forget to start up again. When you get home, you will need to make a deliberate effort to resume your new eating and exercise habits.

Detour 4: Life Changes and Sickness

The third detour is not usually as enjoyable as the first two, but it can be equally destructive. Often a significant change, such as a move to a new city, a new job, divorce, or a hospital stay requires that you focus your attention on coping with your new situation. Even if none of the changes directly affects your eating and exercise behaviors, you now have new challenges that seem more important. It becomes difficult to maintain the new habits.

A minor disruption in routine can also become a detour. For example, if your boss asks you to come in early for two weeks, you might give up your daily morning walks and not resume them even after your schedule returns to normal. Stephanie's four-day bout with the flu almost ended her walking routine.

Detour 5: Negative Emotions

Do you remember your score on the Emotional Eating Scale in Chapter 2? If you got high scores, emotional eating not only is a significant reason for your weight gain, but may also be a detour on the path to weight loss. Think about your dieting history. Can you recall a time when you fought with your husband or had an argument with your mother, felt angry, and were tempted to give up? An unpleasant emotion, such as frustration, anger, or depression, especially if it follows conflict with someone who is important to you, can be very disruptive. One study of dieters in a medical center weight loss program found that almost half of the time that a participant gave up, it was right after an emotional upset.[105] For a more detailed discussion of how to cope with negative emotions without eating, see my book *Emotional Eating: What You Need to Know Before Starting Another Diet*.[106]

Detour 6: Plateaus

Regardless of how conscientious you are, sooner or later you will hit a plateau where your weight remains stable for weeks. You feel increasingly frustrated each time you get on the scale and there is no improvement. It is very easy to get discouraged and assume that it is hopeless. Since your effort isn't getting you anywhere, why bother? The methods that require more effort usually go first, then your weight starts to increase, and pretty soon you give up altogether.

How many of the six detours have you encountered? While the holiday season happens once a year, several of the detours like negative emotions and social pressure can be frequent occurrences, while others like sickness and major life changes occur less often. Regardless of the frequency, if you plan ahead, you will be able to encounter these situations without getting sidetracked. Let's start with what goes on inside your head when you come to a detour.

Thinking About Lapses

In Chapter 5 you examined, and hopefully changed, much of your thinking about dieting. Recall the first negative thought that was described: Dieting is like a light switch—you are either on or off a diet. The same kind of negative thinking can take you from a detour to a relapse. For example, if you have overeaten and underexercised during a vacation, do you think that you've "blown" your diet and give up? Instead, it's helpful to make a distinction between lapse and relapse.

A lapse is an episode (like a week's vacation) where you didn't follow your rules regarding eating or exercise. A lapse is a mistake which, if not corrected, will lead to a relapse. On the other hand, a relapse is a complete return to your behaviors before you started. Any of the detours can cause a lapse, which does not have to progress to a complete relapse. Instead, when you experience a lapse, you could view it as a reasonable error that can be prevented in the future with a little planning. When you have successfully coped with several detours, the likelihood of relapse will decrease and you'll have more self-confidence when you encounter the next detour.

A second type of unhelpful thinking is to assume that the lapse was the result of an inadequacy in your personality, rather than an unfortunate but reasonable response to the circumstances. For example, most people in the midst of a move to a new city find that many of their established routines don't survive the move. If you were in the habit of reading the morning newspaper every day, but stopped after your move, you would not attribute this change to a flaw in your personality. You would recognize that the change in circumstances was the cause. The same is true for eating and exercise habits. Instead of feeling bad, figure out how to reestablish the habits, and develop a plan to avoid similar lapses in the future.

The Path from Detour to Relapse

Now, if you've avoided the unhelpful thinking that can come with a lapse, you can look backward to identify each of the steps that led from the detour to your lapse. For each of the six detours, the descriptions in this chapter should help you figure out what happened. If your husband is participating, get his input. Describe the lapse (without all-or-nothing thinking and self-blame), tell him what you think the sequence of events leading to the lapse might have been, and see if he has any observations. By identifying the sequence of events that starts with a detour, becomes a lapse, and if not corrected, results in a relapse, you will be able to recognize when you are heading down this destructive path. The earlier in the sequence you do this, the easier it is to stop.

After you have figured out the steps leading to the lapse, the next step is to develop plans for coping. For predictable detours (vacations, Christmas parties) you will know ahead of time what to do. For unpredictable detours (sickness, social pressures), once you recognize that you've been detoured, you will be able to retrace your steps to prevent it from becoming a full-blown relapse. Several strategies that have worked for my patients are the following:

1.   Intensify your self-monitoring. Reread Chapter 6. If you've let it slip, start self-monitoring again. If you have been self-monitoring your eating, but not your activity, start recording your activity. If you think it would help, show your daily records to your husband.

2.   Review the relevant parts of Chapters 11 and 12. Find the behaviors that you need to change and ask for your husband's help. For example, before a Christmas party reread the section on parties and social events with your husband and plan what you will do at the party. If your weight has plateaued, can you ask him to

notice and compliment you for your efforts even though your weight hasn't changed?

3.   Write a new reward contract, with a really desirable reward for making the necessary changes. Perhaps you could be rewarded with a weekend away with your husband in January if you can maintain your eating and exercise habits throughout the holiday season.

4.   Use a plateau to consolidate your gains. After you have lost some weight, you will need to get accustomed to your new, lower weight. Family and friends will comment on your weight loss, some people may treat you differently, and it may take some time to become comfortable with your body. Instead of getting discouraged during a plateau, use the time to adjust to your new weight.

Relapse Prevention—The Road to Permanent Weight Control

When she called, Stephanie was in the midst of a lapse which was about to become a relapse. During our phone conversation she decided to keep her appointment for the following day. When I met with her, we discussed much of the information in this chapter. She seemed relieved to learn that detours are inevitable, and having a lapse is not a sign of personal weakness. We reviewed the detours she had encountered, and considered alternative responses she might have made. I gave her a Relapse Prevention Plan and suggested that she get her husband's help completing it.

The next week she resumed her weight loss. Stephanie showed me the Relapse Prevention Plan that she had developed with her husband's help. In addition to plans for coping with social pressure and sickness in the future, they started to talk about the vacation they had planned for the following month. They anticipated eating most of their meals in restaurants so Stephanie was concerned about maintaining her low-fat diet. Her husband agreed not to order dessert when they were eating together and to take responsibility for asking the waitress not to bring bread and butter. They also agreed to go for a walk after dinner every day. Instead of becoming a relapse, Stephanie's detour and lapse were just a temporary interruption in her progress toward permanent weight control.

Developing Your Relapse Prevention Plan

If he is participating, ask your husband to read the letter below, then together work on the Relapse Prevention Plan. This plan will detail how both of you will respond to detours that may occur in the future. If your husband isn't participating, you can still use the Relapse Prevention Plan by yourself so that you will be able to recognize the early signs of a lapse, and prevent it from becoming a relapse. Leave the sections for the husband blank, but fill in your potential detours, what you can do to avoid lapses, and how you will reward yourself for success.

A Note for Your Husband

Dear Husband,

Research shows that a large number of successful dieters regain the weight that they worked so hard to lose. Usually dieting relapses are not the result of personal inadequacies. Instead, an event like a holiday dinner or vacation acts as a detour by disrupting the dieter's routine. The new eating and exercise habits are dropped, but this can be a temporary lapse if she resumes her new habits. Unfortunately, many dieters give up after a lapse and go back to unhealthy eating and underexercising. This is a relapse. You can help ensure that, when your wife has a temporary lapse, it does not become a relapse.

Since all dieters will face detours, your wife is going to ask for your help in developing a Relapse Prevention Plan (Box 29). The first part of the plan is to figure out in advance situations that are likely to create a detour on the road to successful weight loss. You can help her identify these situations, develop methods for dealing with them *before* they occur, and reward each other for successfully avoiding relapse. If you would like a more detailed explanation of relapse prevention, feel free to read the whole chapter.

Box 29. Relapse Prevention Plan

Using Detours 1–6 as a guideline, the following situations have been identified as potential causes of a lapse in eating and exercise habits:

1. _____   6. _____

2. _____   7. _____

3. _____   8. _____

4. _____   9. _____

5. _____   10. _____

When either the husband or the wife suspects that a

detour is leading to a lapse, he or she will raise the issue with the other and describe specific behaviors that suggest a lapse. The husband and the wife will discuss the lapse, and implement the following strategies:

The husband will:

1. _____

2. _____

3. _____

The wife will intensify self-monitoring by:

1. _____

2. _____

3. _____

When the detour has been successfully avoided, or the lapse arrested so that previously established eating and exercise habits are resumed, the husband and the wife will reward each other by:

1. _____

2. _____

_____   _____
Wife   Husband

_____
Date

Is Your Marriage Making You Healthy and Happy?

It's time to review your progress so far, keeping in mind that the different aspects of permanent weight control are not likely to proceed at the same pace. How have you been doing? Are there a few methods that you've put off trying, or ruled out as being impractical? Were there any that you tried a few times, but abandoned before it became a habit? Remember that some behavior changes are more difficult than others, but permanent weight control is a lifelong process. If you persist, you will make enough progress with the methods you have been using so that you can return to the ones you avoided earlier. Allow yourself to feel satisfaction for the changes that you have made; you'll have more self-confidence when it comes to tackling the methods that you've been avoiding.

You will have your good days and your bad days, but permanent weight control is possible if you persist. Take a long-term perspective. You are going to be with your body for the rest of your life, so you need to be good to it and take care of it. The Recipe will help you lose weight and, along the way, improve communication and get closer to your husband. Keep at it.

References

[1]See, for example: Berscheid, E., Walster, E., & Bohrnstedt, G. (November 1973). The happy American body: A survey report. *Psychology Today,* pp. 119–131; and Striegel-Moore, R. H., Silberstein, L. R., & Rodin, J. (1986). Toward an understanding of risk factors for bulimia. *American Psychologist, 41,* 246–263.

[2]Ganley, R. M. (1989). Emotion and eating in obesity: A review of the literature. *International Journal of Eating Disorders, 8,* 343–361.

[3]Hill, A. J., Weaver, C. F. L., & Blundell, J. E. (1991). Food craving, dietary restraint and mood. *Appetite, 17,* 187–197.

[4]Weingarten, H. P. & Elston, D. (1991). Food cravings in a college population. *Appetite, 17,* 167–175.

[5]Glucksman, M. L., Rand, C. S. W., & Stunkard, A. J. (1978). Psychodynamics of obesity. *Journal of the American Academy of Psychoanalysis, 6,* 103–115.

[6]For a review of much of this research see: Striegel-Moore, R. H., Silberstein, L. R., & Rodin, J. (1986). Toward an understanding of risk factors for bulimia. *American Psychologist, 41,* 246–263.

[7]Marino, D. D. & King, J. C. (1980). Nutritional concerns during adolescence. *Pediatric Clinics of North America, 27,* 125–139.

[8]Black, D. R., Gleser, L. J., & Kooyers, K. J. (1990). A meta-analytic evaluation of couples weight-loss programs. *Health Psychology, 9,* 330–347.

[9]Barinaga, M. (1995). "Obese" protein slims mice. *Science, 269,* 475–476.

[10]Burros, M. (July 17, 1994). More Americans tipping the scales. *San Francisco Examiner,* p. A-8.

[11]Bouchard, C. (1995). Genetic influences on body weight and shape. In K. D. Brownell & C. G. Fairburn (Eds.), *Eating disorders and obesity: A comprehensive handbook.* New York: Guilford.

[12]National Task Force on the Prevention and Treatment of Obesity. (1996). Long-term pharmacotherapy in the management of obesity. *Journal of the American Medical Association, 276,* 1907–1915.

[13]Klem, M. L. (1996). Lessons from successful losers. *The Weight Control Digest, 6,* 553, 561-562.

[14]Andres, R. (1995). Body weight and age. In K. D. Brownell & C. G. Fairburn (Eds.), *Eating disorders and obesity: A comprehensive handbook.* New York: Guilford.

[15]McCarty, B. (1992). Fat vs. Muscle. *The Weight Control Digest, 2,* p. 214.

[16]National Academy of Sciences, National Research Council. (1989). *Diet and health: Implications for reducing chronic disease risk.* Washington, D.C.: National Academy Press.

[17]Curb, J. D. & Marcus, E. B. (1991). Body fat and obesity in Japanese Americans. *American Journal of Clinical Nutrition, 53,* 1552S–1555S.

[18]Eric Bromberg quoted in: Stacey, M. (1994). *Consumed: Why Americans love, hate, and fear food.* New York: Touchstone, p. 201.

[19]Arnow, B., Kenardy, J., & Agras, W. S. (1995). The emotional eating scale: The development of a measure to assess coping with negative affect by eating. *International Journal of Eating Disorders, 18,* 79–90.

[20]Grilo, C. M., Shiffman, S., & Wing, R. R. (1989). Relapse crises and coping among dieters. *Journal of Consulting and Clinical Psychology, 57,* 488–495.

[21]Blair, A. J., Lewis, V. J., & Booth, D. A. (1990). Does emotional eating interfere with success in attempts at weight control? *Appetite, 15,* 151–157.

[22]Steinfeld, J. D. (1995). Weight management during pregnancy. *The Weight Control Digest, 5,* 435–436.

[23]Moore, B. J. & Greenwood, M. R. C. (1995). Pregnancy and weight gain. In K. D. Brownell & C. G. Fairburn (Eds.), *Eating disorders and obesity: A comprehensive handbook.* New York: Guilford.

[24]Dewey, K. G., Heining, M. J., & Nommsen, L. A. (1993). Maternal weight loss patterns during prolonged lactation. *American Journal of Clinical Nutrition. 58,* 162–166.

[25]Ohlin, A. & Rossner, S. (1996). Factors related to body weight changes during and after pregnancy: The Stockholm pregnancy and weight development study. *Obesity Research, 4,* 271.

[26]Klesges, R. C. (1995). Cigarette smoking and body weight. In K. D. Brownell and C. G. Fairburn (Eds.), *Eating disorders and obesity: A comprehensive handbook.* New York: Guilford.

[27]Klesges, R. C. (1994). How cigarette smoking and weight are related. *The Weight Control Digest, 4,* 361, 364–366.

[28]Doherty, K., Militello, F. S., Kinnunen, T., & Garvey, A. J. (1996). Nicotine gum dose and weight gain after smoking cessation. *Journal of Consulting and Clinical Psychology, 64,* 799–807.

[29]Stuart, R. B. & Jacobson, B. (1987). *Weight, sex and marriage: A delicate balance.* New York: Norton.

[30]John Updike was interviewed in *The New York Times* by Clyde Haberman on March 6, 1996 (pp. B1, B4).

[31]McCarty, B. (1992). Fat vs. Muscle. *The Weight Control Digest, 2,* 214. This difference is not just a random whim of nature. Women naturally have a higher percentage of body fat which is necessary for reproduction. Since fat requires fewer calories than muscle, a woman needs less to maintain her weight.

[32]Stuart, R. B. & Jacobson, B. (1987). *Weight, sex and marriage: A delicate balance.* New York: Norton.

[33]Klem, M. L. (1996). Lessons from successful losers. *Weight Control Digest, 6,* 553, 561–562.

[34]The rules for communication presented in this chapter were adapted from Dr. Gottman's book, *Why marriages succeed or fail: What you can learn from the breakthrough research to make your marriage last.* New York: Simon & Schuster, 1994.

[35]Black, D. R., Gleser, L. J., & Kooyers, K. J. (1990). A meta-analytic evaluation of couples weight-loss programs. *Health Psychology, 9,* 330–347.

[36]Rand, C. S. W., Kuldu, J. M., & Robbins, L. (1982). Surgery for obesity and marital quality. *Journal of the American Medical Association, 247,* 1419–1422.

[37]Black, D. R. & Threlfall, W. E. (1989). Partner weight status and subject weight loss: Implications for cost-effective programs and public health. *Addictive Behaviors, 14,* 279–289.

[38]Brownell, K. D. & Rodin, J. (1994). The dieting maelstrom: Is it possible and advisable to lose weight? *American Psychologist, 49,* 781–791.

[39]Lowe, M. R. (1993). The effects of dieting on eating behavior: A three-factor model. *Psychological Bulletin, 114,* 100–121.

[40]Stunkard, A. J. (1958). The management of obesity. *New York State Journal of Medicine, 58,* 79–87.

[41]Rating the diets. (June 1993). *Consumer Reports,* 353–357.

[42]Schachter, S. (1982). Recidivism and self-cure of smoking and obesity. *American Psychologist, 37,* 436–444.

[43]Polivy, J., Heatherton, T. F., & Herman, C. P. (1988). Self-esteem, restraint, and eating behavior. *Journal of Abnormal Psychology, 97,* 354–356.

[44]Stacy, M. (1994). *Consumed: Why Americans love, hate and fear food.* New York: Touchstone, pp. 13, 31.

[45]Baumeister, R. (1996). Paper presented at the annual meeting of The American Psychological Association, Toronto.

[46]Baker, R. C. & Kirschenbaum, D. S. (1993). Self-monitoring may be necessary for successful weight control. *Behavior Therapy, 24,* 377–394.

[47]Wifley, D. E. & Rodin, J. (1995). Cultural influences on eating disorders. In K. D. Brownell & C. G. Fairburn, (Eds.), *Eating disorders and obesity: A comprehensive handbook.* New York: Guilford.

[48]Daniels, E. S. (1996). A feminist look at body image. *The Weight Control Digest, 6,* 515–517.

[49]Pi-Sunyer, F. X. (1995). Medical complications of obesity. In K. D. Brownell & C. G. Fairburn (Eds.), *Eating disorders and obesity: A comprehensive handbook.* New York: Guilford.

[50]Blackburn, G. L. (1995). Effects of weight loss on weight-related risk factors. In K. D. Brownell & C. G. Fairburn (Eds.), *Eating disorders and obesity: A comprehensive handbook.* New York: Guilford, p. 406.

[51]Brownell, K. D. & Wadden, T. A. (1991). The heterogeneity of obesity: Fitting treatments to individuals. *Behavior Therapy, 22,* 153–177.

[52]Bouchard, C. (1995). Genetic influences on body weight and shape. In Brownell, K. D. & Fairburn C. G. (Eds.).

Eating disorders and obesity: A comprehensive handbook. New York: Guilford.

[53]Wilson, G. T. (1996). Acceptance and change in the treatment of eating disorders and obesity. *Behavior Therapy, 27,* 417–439.

[54]Jacobson, N. S. & Christensen, A. (1996). *Integrative couple therapy: Promoting acceptance and change.* New York: Norton, p. 42.

[55]Heavey, C. L., Layne, C., & Christensen, A. (1993). Gender and conflict structure in marital interaction: A replication and extension. *Journal of Consulting and Clinical Psychology, 61,* 16–27.

[56]Heavey, C. L., Christensen, A., & Malamuth, N. M. (1995). The longitudinal impact of demand and withdrawal during marital conflict. *Journal of Consulting and Clinical Psychology, 63,* 797–801.

[57]Ted Huston quoted in Hatfield, E. & Rapson, R. L. (1993). *Love, sex and intimacy: Their psychology, biology, and history.* New York: HarperCollins, p. 154.

[58]See Chapter 5 in Hatfield, E. & Rapson, R. L. (1993). *Love, sex and intimacy: Their psychology, biology, and history.* New York: HarperCollins.

[59]Felitti, V. J. (1993). Childhood sexual abuse, depression, and family dysfunction in adult obese patients: A case control study. *Southern Medical Journal, 86,* 732–736.

[60]Stotland, S. & Zuroff, D. C. (1991). Relations between multiple measures of dieting self-efficacy and weight change in a behavioral weight control program. *Behavior Therapy, 22,* 47–59.

[61]Rosen, J. C., Orosan, P., & Reiter, J. (1995). Cognitive behavior therapy for negative body image in obese women. *Behavior Therapy, 26,* 25–42.

[62]Jacobson, N. S. & Christensen, A. (1996). *Integrative couple therapy: Promoting acceptance and change.* New York: Norton, p. 153.

[63]Masters, W. H., Johnson, V. E., & Kolodny, R. C. (1985).

Human Sexuality (2d Ed.). Boston: Little, Brown, chapter 13.

[64]Hatfield, E., Sprecher, S., Pillemer, J. T., Greenberger, D., & Wexler, P. (1988). Gender differences in what is desired in the sexual relationship. *Journal of Psychology and Human Sexuality, 1,* 39–52.

[65]Felitti, V. J. (1991). Long-term medical consequences of incest, rape, and molestation. *Southern Medical Journal, 84,* 328–331.

[66]King, T. K., Clark, M. M., & Pera, V. (1996). History of sexual abuse and obesity treatment outcome. *Addictive Behavior, 21,* 283–290.

[67]Felitti, V. J. (1993). Childhood sexual abuse, depression, and family dysfunction in adult obese patients: A case control study. *Southern Medical Journal, 86,* 732–736.

[68]DiGiuseppe, R., Tafrate, R., & Eckhardt, C. (1994). Critical issues in the treatment of anger. *Cognitive and Behavioral Practice, 1,* 111–132.

[69]Lerner, H. G. (1986). *The dance of anger: A woman's guide to changing the patterns of intimate relationships.* New York: Perennial.

[70]Spielberger, C. D. (1992). Anger/hostility, heart disease and cancer. Cited in DiGiuseppe, R., Tafrate, R., & Eckhardt, C. (1994). Critical issues in the treatment of anger. *Cognitive and Behavioral Practice, 1,* 111–132.

[71]Rubin, T. I. (1970). *The angry book.* New York: Collier.

[72]Siegel, J. M. (1992). Anger and cardiovascular health. In H. S. Friedman (Ed.), *Hostility coping and health.* Washington, D.C.: American Psychological Association, pp. 49–64.

[73]The distinction between anger and annoyance is based on work by Albert Ellis, especially *How to live with and without anger.* New York: Readers' Digest Press, 1977.

[74]Weiss, L., Katzman, M., & Wolchik, S. (1985). *Treating bulimia: A psychoeducational approach.* New York: Pergamon.

[75]Martin, J. (July 19, 1996). When "No, thanks" isn't enough. *San Francisco Chronicle*, p. D–18.

[76]Tavris, C. (1982). *Anger: The misunderstood emotion*. New York: Simon & Schuster.

[77]Averill, J. R. (1983). Studies on anger and aggression: Implications for theories on emotion. *American Psychologist, 38*, 1145–1160.

[78]For example: Marshall, J. R. (1977). The removal of a psychosomatic symptom: Effects on the marriage. *Family Process, 16,* 273–280; Minuchin, S., Rossman, B., & Baker, L. (1978). *Psychosomatic families*. Cambridge: Harvard University Press; and Selvini-Palazzoli, M. (1978). *Self-starvation: From the intrapsychic to the transpersonal approach to anorexia nervosa*. New York: Jason Aronson.

[79]Weisz, G. & Bucher, B. (1980). Involving husbands in the treatment of obesity—Effects on weight loss, depression and marital satisfaction. *Behavior Therapy, 11,* 643–650.

[80]Power, D. & Abramson, E. E. (July 1997). *Relationship of weight loss to marital adjustment*. Paper presented at the Fifth European Congress of Psychology, Dublin, Ireland.

[81]Stuart, R. B. & Jacobson, B. (1987). *Weight, sex and marriage: A delicate balance*. New York: Norton, p. 71.

[82]Brownell, K. D. & Wadden, T. A. (1991). The heterogeneity of obesity: Fitting treatments to individuals. *Behavior Therapy, 22,* 153–177.

[83]The Center for Science in the Public Interest bought dishes from: T.G.I. Friday's, Denny's, El Torito, Chi-Chi's, Chili's, Olive Garden, and Big Boy. Three quarters of the items from the healthy menus met the 30% fat calorie criterion. See: Burros, M. (November 30, 1995). Low-fat menus fare well in a study of restaurants. *New York Times*, A-17.

[84]Two low-fat bestsellers are: *In the kitchen with Rosie* by Rosie

Daley (Knopf) and *Eat more, Weigh less* by Dean Ornish (HarperCollins). There are many others; just try to avoid cookbooks that are too spartan, or make eating a medical exercise rather than a pleasurable activity.

[85]Blundell, J. E. & Hill, A. J. (1993). Binge eating: Psychobiological mechanisms. In Fairburn, C. G. & Wilson, G. T. (Eds.), *Binge eating: Nature, assessment, and treatment.* New York: Guilford.

[86]Leary, W. E. (September 6, 1995). Recipe for weight gain: Alcohol and fatty foods. *New York Times*, B–6.

[87]Hager, D. L. (1993). Breakfast: To have or have not! *Weight Control Digest, 3,* 225–226.

[88]Shapiro, L. (December 9, 1994). A food lover's guide to fat. *Newsweek,* 52–55, 58–60.

[89]O'Neill, M. (February 8, 1995). So it may be true after all: Eating pasta makes you fat. *New York Times*, A–1, B–7.

[90]Kolata, G. (April 25, 1995). Benefit of standard low-fat diet is doubted. *New York Times*, B7–B8.

[91]See: Abramson, E. E. (1977). *Behavioral approaches to weight control.* New York: Springer.

[92]Grilo, C. M., Wilfley, D. E., & Brownell, K. D. (1992). Physical activity and weight control: Why is the link so strong. *Weight Control Digest, 2,* 153, 157–160.

[93]Brody, J. E. (March 8, 1995). Personal health: Studies warn that women are not doing all they can to reduce the risk of heart disease. *The New York Times,* B–7.

[94]Blair, S. N., Kohl, H. W., Paffenbarger, R. S., Clark, D. G., Cooper, K. H., & Gibbons, L. W. (1989). Physical fitness and all-cause mortality: A prospective study of healthy men and women. *Journal of the American Medical Association, 262,* 2395–2401.

[95]Brody, J. E. (February 8, 1995). Personal health: How to experience the health benefits of regular exercise without working up a sweat. *The New York Times,* B–5.

[96]For example, see: Doyne, E. J., Ossip-Klein, D. J.,

Bowman, E. D., Osborn, K. M., McDougall-Wilson, B., & Neimeyer, R. A. (1987). Running versus weight lifting in the treatment of depression. *Journal of Consulting and Clinical Psychology, 55,* 748–754.

[97]Brownell, K. D. (1995). Exercise in the treatment of obesity. In Brownell, K. D. & Fairburn, C. G. (Eds.), *Eating disorders and obesity: A comprehensive handbook.* New York: Guilford.

[98]Kayman, S., Bruvold, W., & Stern, J. S. (1990). Maintenance and relapse after weight loss in women: Behavioral aspects. *American Journal of Clinical Nutrition, 52,* 800–807.

[99]Tucker, A. & Bagwell, M. (1991). Television viewing and obesity in adult females. *American Journal of Public Health, 81,* 1908–1911.

[100]Ravussin, E. (1995). Energy expenditure and body weight. In Brownell, K. D. & Fairburn, C. G. (Eds.), *Eating disorders and obesity: A comprehensive handbook.* New York: Guilford.

[101]Perri, M. G., Martin, A. D., Leermakers, E. A., Sears, S. F., & Notelovitz, M. (1997). Effects of group- versus home-based exercise in the treatment of obesity. *Journal of Consulting and Clinical Psychology, 65,* 278–285.

[102]For a summary see: Anderson, R. (1997). Physical activity and health: The U.S. Surgeon General's Report. *The Weight Control Digest, 7,* 612–613.

[103]Boutelle, K. N., Kirschenbaum, D. S., Baker, R. C., & Mitchell, M. E. (November 1996). How to minimize weight gain during the holidays: Self-monitor very consistently. Paper presented at the annual meeting of the Association for Advancement of Behavior Therapy, New York.

[104]Kirschenbaum, D. S. (November 1996). Preventing weight gain during the holidays: The critical role of self-monitoring. Paper presented at the annual meeting of the

Association for Advancement of Behavior Therapy, New York.

[105]Grilo, C. M., Schiffman, S., & Wing, R. R. (1989). Relapse crises and coping among dieters. *Journal of Consulting and Clinical Psychology, 57,* 488–495.

[106]Abramson, E. E. (1998). *Emotional eating: What you need to know before starting another diet.* San Francisco, Jossey-Bass.

For information about workshops or lectures write:

Dr. Edward Abramson
Dept. of Psychology
California State University, Chico
Chico, CA 95929

Please include a self-addressed stamped envelope.

Parenting Advice

__Baby: An Owner's Manual

$14.00US/$17.00CAN

By Bud Zukow, M.D. and Nancy Kaneshiro   1-57566-055-5

Dr. Zukow has been fielding parents' most common (and not-so-common) pediatric questions for more than 30 years. From ground zero through the end of the first year, this wise, witty, indispensible book provides answers and practical tips for your most pressing problems.

__How to Get the Best Public Education for Your Child

A Practical Parent's Guide for the 1990's $4.50US/$5.50CAN

By Carol A. Ryan & Paula Sline with Barbara Lagowski   0-8217-4038-5

Here is an insider's perspective combining general information with specific advice. The book includes how to select the best school for your child, how to judge your child's progress, and how to evaluate their teachers. Written by two authors with over 40 years of combined experience in education, this guide will help children fulfill their potential.

__Stepparenting

Everything You Need to Know to Make it Work $13.00US/$16.00CAN

By Jeanette Lofas, CSW, with Dawn B. Sova   1-57566-113-6

Practical, current advice for dealing with the many baffling issues that beset today's stepfamilies. From dating to remarriage, from stepsibling rivalry to joint custody, here is an invaluable resource for coping with today's most complex challenges. Discover the techniques, tools, and strategies that break through the barriers and lead to familial harmony.

Call toll free **1-888-345-BOOK** to order by phone or use this coupon to order by mail.

Name _____

Address _____

City _____ State _____ Zip _____

Please send me the books I have checked above.

I am enclosing $_____

Plus postage and handling* $_____

Sales tax (in New York and Tennessee) $_____

Total amount enclosed $_____

*Add $2.50 for the first book and $.50 for each additional book.

Send check or money order (no cash or CODs) to:

Kensington Publishing Corp., 850 Third Avenue, New York, NY 10022

Prices and Numbers subject to change without notice.

All orders subject to availability.

Check out our website at **www.kensingtonbooks.com**